ECG
for Nurses

Tarika Sharma
MSc Cardiological/CTVS Nursing, BSc (Hons) Nursing (AIIMS, New Delhi)
Faculty
College of Nursing Institute of Liver and Biliary Sciences
New Delhi

Urvashi Sharma
MSc Cardiological/CTVS Nursing, BSc (Hons) Nursing (AIIMS, New Delhi)
Faculty
KGMU College of Nursing
King George's Medical University
Lucknow

Foreword
Manju Vatsa

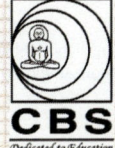

CBS Publishers & Distributors Pvt Ltd
• New Delhi • Bengaluru • Chennai • Kochi • Kolkata • Mumbai
• Hyderabad • Nagpur • Patna • Pune • Vijayawada

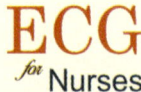

ECG
for Nurses

ISBN: 978-93-89261-88-2

Copyright © Publishers

Reprint: 2021

First Edition: 2020

Published by **Satish Kumar Jain** and produced by **Varun Jain** for

CBS Publishers & Distributors Pvt Ltd

4819/XI Prahlad Street, 24 Ansari Road, Daryaganj, New Delhi 110 002, India.

Ph: +91-11-23289259, 23266861, 23266867   Website: www.cbspd.com

Fax: 011-23243014

e-mail: delhi@cbspd.com; cbspubs@airtelmail.in.

Corporate Office: 204 FIE, Industrial Area, Patparganj, Delhi 110 092

Ph: +91-11-4934 4934   Fax: 4934 4935

e-mail: feedback@cbspd.com; bhupesharora@cbspd.com

Branches

- **Bengaluru:** Seema House 2975, 17th Cross, K.R. Road, Banasankari 2nd Stage, Bengaluru 560 070, Karnataka
  Ph: +91-80-26771678/79   Fax: +91-80-26771680
  e-mail: bangalore@cbspd.com

- **Chennai:** 7, Subbaraya Street, Shenoy Nagar, Chennai 600 030, Tamil Nadu
  Ph: +91-44-26680620, 26681266   Fax: +91-44-42032115
  e-mail: chennai@cbspd.com

- **Kochi:** 68/1534, 35, 36-Power House Road, Opp. KSEB, Cochin-682018, Kochi, Kerala
  Ph: +91-484-4059061-65   Fax: +91-484-4059065
  e-mail: kochi@cbspd.com

- **Kolkata:** 6/B, Ground Floor, Rameswar Shaw Road, Kolkata-700 014, West Bengal
  Ph: +91-33-22891126, 22891127, 22891128
  e-mail: kolkata@cbspd.com

- **Mumbai:** PWD Shed, Gala No. 25/26, Ramchandra Bhatt Marg, Next to J.J. Hospital Gate No. 2, Opp. Union Bank of India, Noor Baug, Mumbai-400009
  Ph: +91-22-66661880/89   Fax: +91-22-24902342
  e-mail: mumbai@cbspd.com

Representatives

Hyderabad	+91-9885175004	**Patna**	+91-9334159340
Pune	+91-9623451994	**Vijayawada**	+91-9000660880

Printed at: Goyal Offset Works Pvt. Ltd.

Dedication

We are extremely grateful to our beloved teacher **Dr G Rachel Andrews** who has been the guiding light for both of us in shaping our thoughts and dreams in the field of Cardiac Nursing. We have been constantly looking up to her for endless inspiration in this journey.

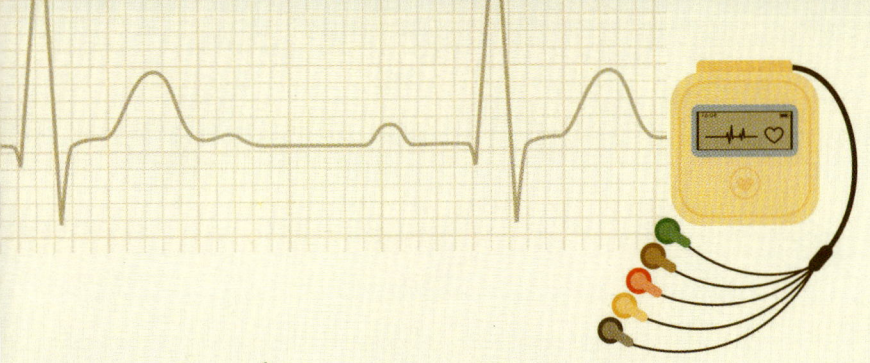

Foreword

I am delighted to write a foreword to the first edition of this valuable text on "ECG for Nurses", presented by Ms Tarika Sharma and Ms Urvashi Sharma, two bright young nursing faculty members; both of whom I have had the pleasure of mentoring. Their commitment and dedication to transform and improve the delivery of nursing care is indeed evidenced through this valuable contribution. The text is targeted for the nursing students and professionals, in the care of cardiac and critical care patients.

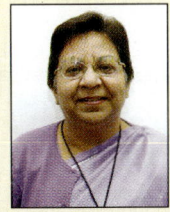

ECG is the most important diagnostic measure to identify the lethal heart rhythms. Nurses are the first line professionals and directly linked to the patient care. Identification of the life-threatening arrhythmias is mandatory for them to take immediate necessary action.

This is probably the first book in India on ECG, by the nurses, for the nurses. The text is presented in a simple language with plenty of visuals to make it easy and interesting for the readers. Nursing students at the undergraduate as well advanced levels and nursing professionals will find it useful to understand the ECG step by step and in managing patients in the clinical setting.

This book aims to improve and upgrade ECG knowledge of the professional nurses and nurse practitioners. I trust that this book will become a useful compendium for nurses working in the cardiac care unit, critical care unit and emergency department, and will contribute to improve patient care in these units.

Dr Manju Vatsa BSN, MSN, MPhil, PhD
Former Principal
College of Nursing, AIIMS, New Delhi
Founder President
Indian Association of Neonatal Nurses

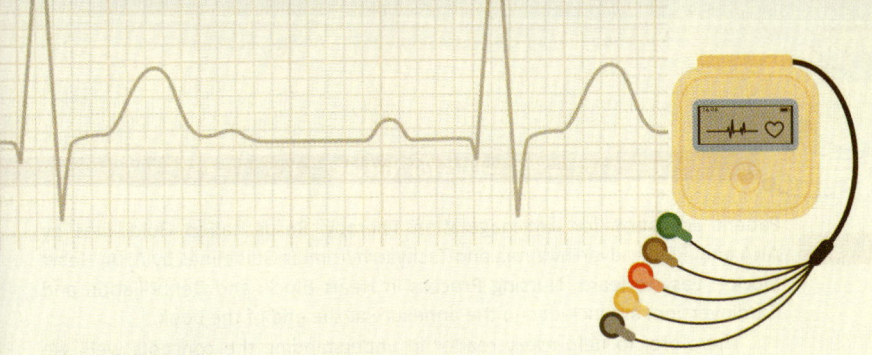

Preface

It gives us immense pleasure to present the first edition of **"ECG for Nurses"** for Nursing Students and Nursing Professionals.

Out of many diagnostic investigations, ECG is most important for the Nurses. Since Nurses are the first line caregivers, they need to have sound knowledge of ECG. Especially Nurses working in units like cardiac care unit, critical care unit, emergency, etc. where immediate prominent action can save the life of the patient, it is necessary for them to understand the various aspects of the hemodynamic monitoring.

The motivation behind for writing this book came through our student's queries and zeal to learn ECG. Considering the enthusiasm of nursing students towards learning and developing the skills for interpreting ECG, we aimed to create a compendium which is easy to understand, able to answer all the queries, and clear the concepts while maintaining the interest of the students.

We have adopted a tabular layout to present the content. The step wise step concept has been used in the table, so that the content can be understood, absorbed and retained by learners. The QRS morphology in each lead is explained in detail but, at the same time in an easy manner. Details of augmented and bipolar limb leads are explained with separate diagrams for each step. Arrhythmias are also explained using step by step approach in tables, so that none of the important aspects is missed. The self-explanatory colored diagrams of the book add clarity to the content.

The nursing process is the backbone of the nursing profession. Alone understanding the ECG will not solve the purpose, until and unless nursing interventions for the same are not understood. Keeping the same in mind, nursing process has been included in the book to reinforce the role of nurses in the management of patients presenting with arrhythmias and heart blocks.

Practice questions at the end of each chapter will help the students to self-assess themselves and these practice questions will help them in various competitive exams.

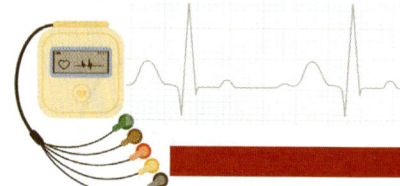

Patient education for Anticoagulation Therapy, Resuscitation Guidelines by AHA and IRC, Bradyarrhythmia and Tachyarrhythmias Guidelines by AHA, Heart block – Easy to learn, Nursing Process in Heart Block, and Defibrillation and Cardioversion, are included in the annexure at the end of the book.

Therefore, to help every reader in understanding the concepts well, we have prepared brief videos on ECG that cover basic to advanced information. We are sure the videos will help the readers.

Suggestions and comments are welcomed by the readers about the book.

We wish all success and blessings to our readers.

Tarika Sharma
Urvashi Sharma

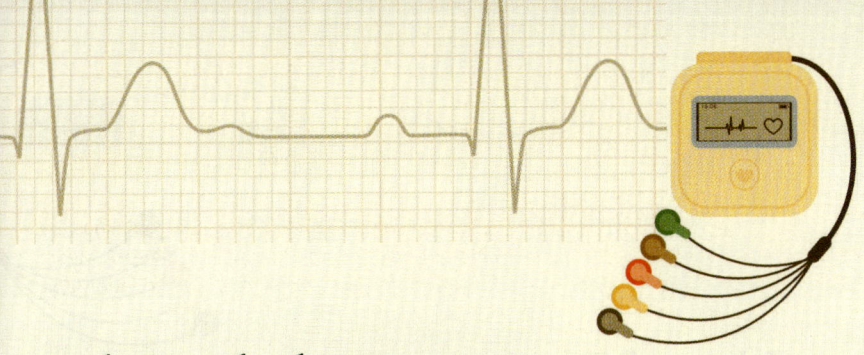

Acknowledgements

At the outset we would like to thank Almighty God with a humble heart for providing us the strength to take up this work and complete it with his grace. It's been said that:

If you can dream it, you can do it!

—*Walt Disney*

Writing a book was a dream for young authors like us which became reality because of the support we got from many people. We owe a huge gratitude to all of them. We would like to express a heartfelt thanks to our teachers who laid the foundation of shaping our career.

There are no words to thank our families who have always been a pillar of strength to both of us in all our endeavors.

We extend our sincere thanks to Dr Manju Vatsa, Former Principal, College of Nursing, AIIMS, New Delhi for writing the Foreword in our book.

This book could not be shaped the way it is without the expert comments of all the reviewers. We would like to thank each of our reviewers for their contribution in this book.

We would like to thank **Mr Satish Kumar Jain** (Chairman) and **Mr Varun Jain** (Managing Director), M/s CBS Publishers and Distributors Pvt Ltd for providing us the platform in bringing out the book. We have no words to describe the role, efforts, inputs and initiatives undertaken by **Mr Bhupesh Arora,** (Vice President - Publishing and Marketing, PGMEE and Nursing Division) for helping and motivating us.

We sincerely thank the entire CBS team for bringing the book colourful with utmost care and presentation. I thank Dr Mrinalini Bakshi (Editorial Head and Content Strategist) for her editorial support and Ms Nitasha Arora (Production Head & Content Strategist), Dr Anju Dhir (Senior Scientific Coordinator/ Editor), Mr Nitish Dubey (Senior Editor) and all the production team members Mr Ashutosh Pathak, Mr Chaman Lal, Mr Prakash Gaur, Mr Phool Kumar, Mr Bunty Kashyap, Ms Tahira Parveen, Ms Babita Verma, Mr Chander, Mr Raju Sharma, Mr Manoj Chaudhary, Mr Vikram Chaudhary, Mr Manoj Malakar, Mr Arun Kumar and Ms Manorama for devoting laborious hours in designing and typesetting of the book.

Last but not the least we would like to thank our students who also inspired us to write the book with their queries and zeal to learn ECG.

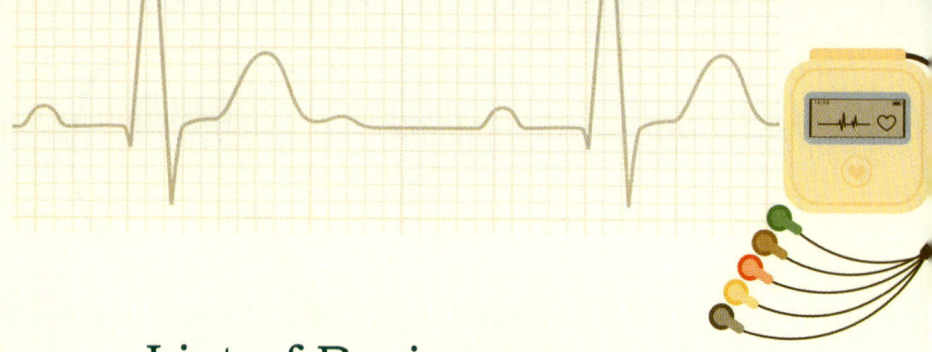

List of Reviewers

- Dr G Rachel Andrews, Former Lecturer, College of Nursing, AIIMS, New Delhi.
- Dr Shashi Mawar, Lecturer, College of Nursing, AIIMS, New Delhi.
- Dr Gopichandran Lakshmanan, Lecturer, College of Nursing, AIIMS, New Delhi.
- Dr Manju Dhandapani, Lecturer, NINE, PGIMER, Chandigarh.
- Ms Smita Das, Lecturer, College of Nursing, AIIMS, New Delhi.
- Ms Shikha Gulia, Tutor, MM College of Nursing, MM University, Mullana, Ambala, Haryana.
- Ms Sarita, Lecturer, College of Nursing, Institute of Liver and Biliary Science (ILBS), New Delhi.
- Dr Koushal Dave, Tutor, College of Nursing, Dr Ram Manohar Lohia Hospital, New Delhi.
- Dr Arun Sood, Senior Consultant Cardiology, Institute of Liver and Biliary Science (ILBS), New Delhi.
- Dr Vikas Thakran, Consultant Interventional Cardiology, Kalra Hospital, New Delhi.
- Ms Divya Sharma, Clinical Quality Improvement Consultant, Alberta Health Services, Canada.
- Dr Karthik T Ponnappant, Consultant Anesthesia, Institute of Liver and Biliary Science (ILBS), New Delhi.
- Dr Pravesh Vishwakarma Associate Professor, Department of Cardiology, King George's Medical University, Lucknow.

Student Reviewers

- Shivam Jaiswar (BSc Nursing, 4th year student)
- Arpita Samridhi (BSc Nursing, 1st year student)
- Prabhat Singh (BSc Nursing, 3rd year student)
- Dharmendra Jaiswal (BSc Nursing, 4th year student)

KGMU College of Nursing, King George's Medical University, Lucknow.

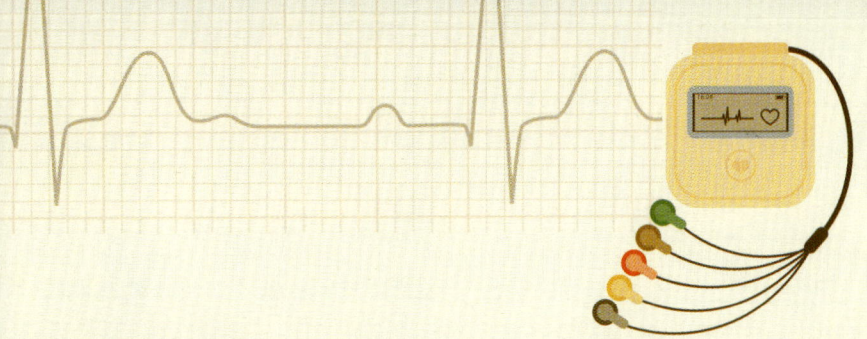

Contents

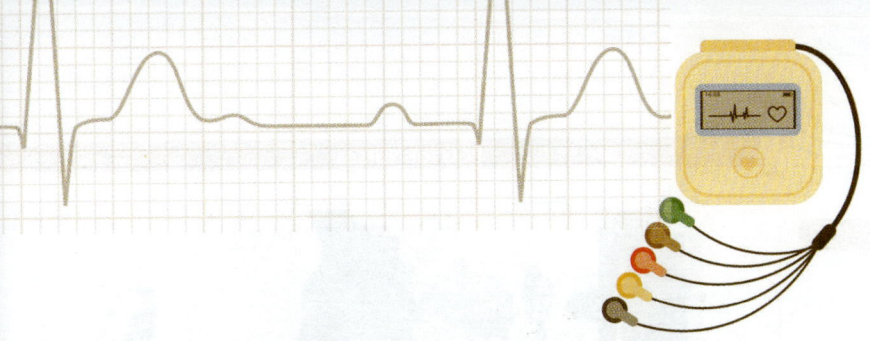

Introduction to Basic ECG

Chapter 1

INTRODUCTION

The word electrocardiograph is derived from Greek word, '*electro + kardio + graph*,' which means, '*electrical activity + heart + to write*, i.e. to record electrical activity of the heart. The knowledge of electrocardiogram (ECG or EKG) is an important aspect for improving the nursing care in a cardiac patient. The prompt and skilled knowledge of identifying changes in ECG makes nurses competent enough to be the part of the cardiac health care team.

ECG is the most valuable, quick and one of the least expensive diagnostic tests that can help the health care professionals to understand many cardiac diseases/disorders at any one time. It is the basic simple test that contains information about a number of cardiac diseases.

Accurate interpretation and understanding of ECG is an important and crucial aspect, needed by a physician and a nurse to approach and treat the patient at right time before occurrence of any hazardous event.

BRIEF HISTORY OF ECG

Willem Einthoven (21 May, 1860 – 29 September 1927), a Dutch physiologist, invented the first practical electrocardiogram in 1903, for which he received a Nobel Prize in medicine, in 1924. **Willem Einthoven** used a string galvanometer for recording ECG and assigned the letters to various deflections as **P, Q, R, S** and **T**, which are still used (Fig. 1.1).

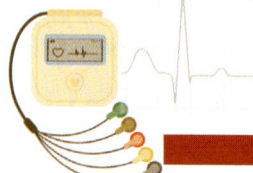

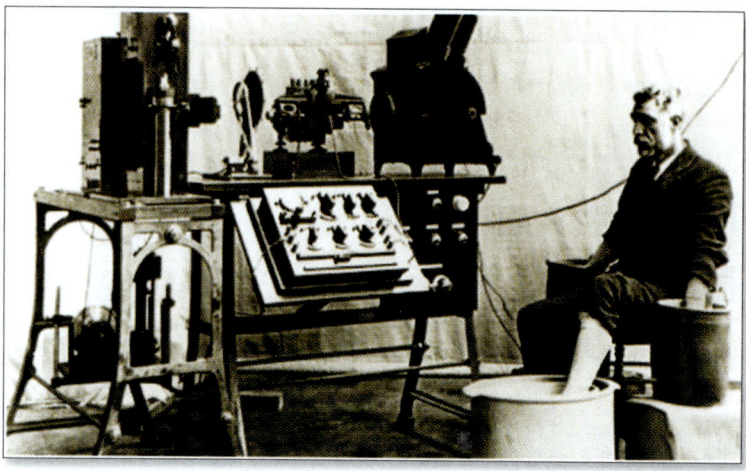

Fig. 1.1 Old string galvanometer electrocardiograph

(**Source:** *AlGhatrif M, Lindsay J. A brief review: history to understand fundamentals of electrocardiography. Journal of community hospital internal medicine perspectives. 2012 Jan 1;2(1):14383*).

DEFINITIONS

Electrocardiogram is the recording of electrical events of the heart using electrodes placed on the skin (12 lead system). It gives a broad picture of the conduction system of the heart, by identifying the minute changes in the electrical activity.

The ECG records the electrical sequence of the heart and gives an information regarding rate, rhythm and the blood flow to cardiac muscles (Fig. 1.2). The normal ECG has P wave, QRS complex, T wave and U wave, where P wave denotes atrial contraction, QRS complex denotes ventricular contraction, T wave

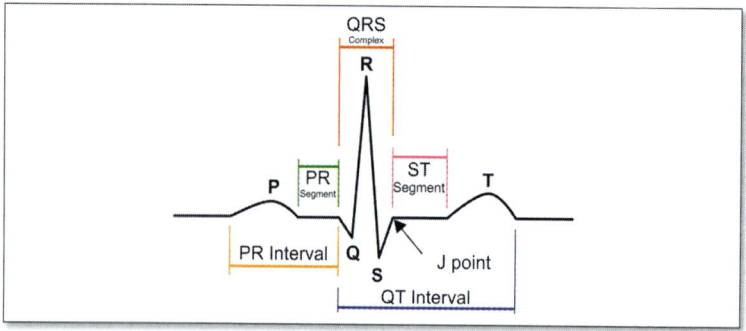

Fig. 1.2 ECG waveform

denotes ventricular repolarization. The U wave is followed by the T wave. The U wave is may not be seen in the ECG due to small size.

In an ECG waveform, there are intervals and segments. **Interval** includes a wave plus segment and **segment** includes a straight line between waves.

Table 1.1 Types of ECG wave forms with their explanations

Waveforms	Explanation	Duration
P wave	Atrial depolarization	≤0.12 sec
QRS wave	Ventricular depolarization	0.06–0.10 sec
T wave	Ventricular repolarization	0.10–0.25 sec
PR interval	Time period from initiation of atrial depolarization to initiation of ventricular depolarization.	0.12 0.20 sec
PR segment	Isoelectric line from end of P wave to onset of QRS, depicting slowing of conduction through atrio-ventricular node. PR segment is baseline or isoelectric line	
J point	J or Junction point is where QRS complex and ST segment meets.	
ST segment	Starts from J point to onset of T wave.	
QT interval	From onset of QRS complex to end of T wave. It represents total time of ventricular depolarization and repolarization.	0.36-0.44 sec (9-11 small boxes)
R-R interval	Interval between two R waves	0.6 – 1.0 sec

Types of ECG forms have been given in Table 1.1.

The **first wave** in ECG is P wave, which is positive, smooth and has a small deflection. P wave represents atrial depolarization (contraction).

The conduction through sinoatrial (SA) node to atrioventricular (AV) node is measured by **PR interval**. The PR interval is from onset of P wave to onset of QRS complex.

The **PR segment** is a straight line which is an isoelectric line starting from end of P wave to the onset of QRS complex.

The **QRS complex** represents ventricular depolarization (contraction). The QRS complex has three waves – Q, R and S wave.

In a QRS complex (Fig. 1.2), the Q wave is the first wave which negative deflection (below isoelctric line) followed by R wave which is first positive wave (above isoelctric line). The next negative deflection is S wave which follows R wave. (for details see in chapter 4)

T wave represents ventricular repolarization (relaxation).

U wave is a positive wave which is one fourth of T wave's amplitude and is seen, occasionally.

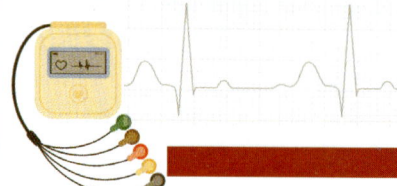
QT interval duration represents total duration of ventricular depolarization and repolarization.

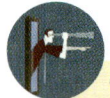

Note --

QT Duration is inversely proportional to heart rate.

QT interval ∝ 1/HR

If HR ↑ses ---------- QT interval ↓ses

If HR ↓ses ---------- QT interval ↑ses

Prolonged QT interval is associated with a risk of cardiac arrhythmias and can provoke Torsades des Pointes, which leads to ventricular fibrillation, thereby causing sudden cardiac death.

ELECTROCARDIOGRAPHS

These are the machines that are used to record ECG. The major component of the machine is *instrumentation amplifier*, which brings voltage difference and amplifies the signal. The machine which is attached to alternating current or AC, is protected against voltage fluctuations by using voltage protection system. The defibrillation protection is also given because ECG leads may be attached to a person who requires defibrillation, therefore the ECG machine needs to be protected from variation in energy source.

Conventionally, the electrocardiograph machines are small portable wheeled carts units with a screen, keyboard (for entering patient's details) and a printer (to print patient's report).

UNDERSTANDING CONDUCTION SYSTEM OF THE HEART

The heart is four chambered muscular organ that pumps blood throughout the body and is located between the lungs in the thoracic cavity (Fig. 1.3).

The heart has mainly two types of cells: **cardiomyocytes** and **cardiac pacemaker cells.**

Cardiomyocytes make up the cardiac muscles, i.e. chambers (atria and ventricles) of the heart. They are interconnected by *intercalated discs* forming junctions (helps to work as a single functional organ) and enable the muscles of heart to shorten and lengthen their fibers, i.e. leads to easier depolarization and repolarization in the myocardium.

The heart is able to act as a single functional coordinated unit because of these junctions and bridges.

The **cardiac pacemaker cells** are the specialized cells which spontaneously initiate the impulses causing beating of a heart.

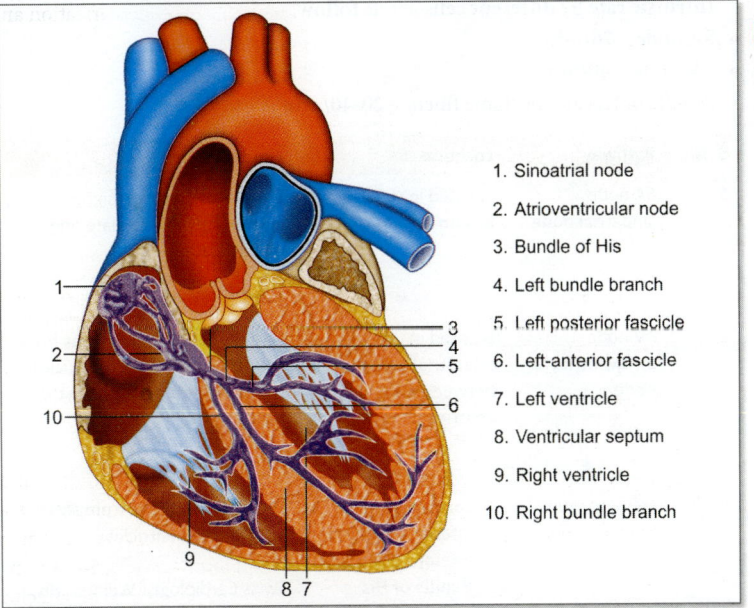

1. Sinoatrial node
2. Atrioventricular node
3. Bundle of His
4. Left bundle branch
5. Left posterior fascicle
6. Left-anterior fascicle
7. Left ventricle
8. Ventricular septum
9. Right ventricle
10. Right bundle branch

Fig. 1.3 Conduction system of the heart

Properties of the Cardiac Pacemaker Cells

- Able to generate and send electrical impulses spontaneously
- Able to receive and respond to the electrical impulses received from the brain
- Able to transfer these electrical impulses from one cell to another cell

Sinoatrial Node

Sinoatrial (SA) node is the **natural pacemaker** of the heart.

Sinoatrial node has the fastest automaticity (means generates impulse at 60 to 100 bpm) compared to AV node (impulse generation rate around 40-50 bpm), bundle of His (impulse rate around 30-40 bpm) and purkinje fibres (around 15-30 bpm), thats why sinoatrial node is considered as natural pacemaker of the heart.

The group of pacemaker cells from the SA node generates an electrical current spontaneously that gives rise to the rhythm and causes contraction of the heart and is responsible for beating of a heart.

The pumping action of the heart can be credited to the rhythm which is determined by this group of pacemaker cells.

Intrinsic rate by different cells are as follow:

- SA node – **70/min**
- AV node – **40/min**
- Bundle of His and purkinje fibers – **20-40/min**

S. No.	Pathway	Location	Function
1.	SA node sinoatrial node	Located in right atrium	Generates electrical signal or impulses to stimulate and contract atria.
	↓		
2.	AV node atrioventricular node	Located in the interatrial septum between atria and ventricles	Screens out rapid impulses from the atria, preventing ventricles from life-threatening arrhythmia
	↓		
3.	Left and right Bundle of His	• Located at the inferior end of the interatrial septum • Bundle of His branches into left and right branches, which run along the interventricular septum	Transmits impulses from AV node to the ventricles. Swiss Cardiologist Wilhelm His, Jr., discovered this specialized muscle fibres in 1893 and therefore named after him.
	↓		
4.	Purkinje fibres	Located in inner ventricular walls of the heart, in the subendocardium space beneath the endocardium	Carry and transmit the impulse from both left and right bundle of His to the ventricles. Specialized conducting fibers, with larger number of mitochondria are therefore able to conduct cardiac action potential more quickly than any other cells in the heart. It helps to conduct synchronized contractions of the ventricles

Left bundle of His further branches into left posterior fascicle and left anterior fascicle. The posterior fascicle, which is actually broad band of fibres, spreads over the posterior and inferior surfaces of the left ventricle, where as anterior fascicle is a narrow band of fibres spreading over the anterior and superior surfaces of the left ventricle (Fig. 1.4).

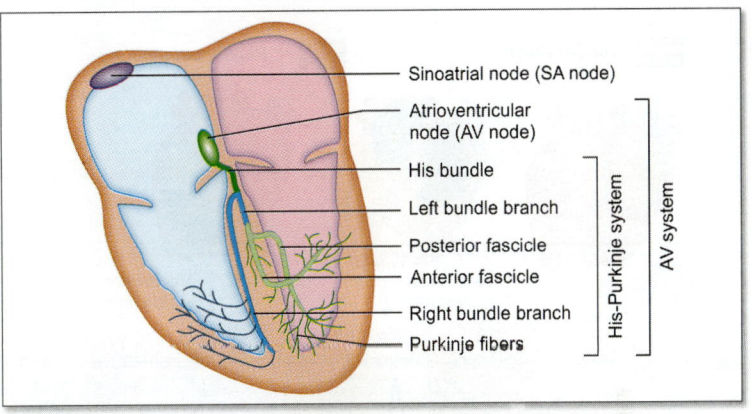

Sinoatrial node (SA node)

Atrioventricular node (AV node)

His bundle

Left bundle branch

Posterior fascicle

Anterior fascicle

Right bundle branch

Purkinje fibers

His-Purkinje system

AV system

Fig. 1.4 Branches of left bundle of His – anterior and posterior fascicle

Purkinje fibres travel across the complete myocardium thickness, thereby activating entire myocardial mass from endocardial to epicardial surface.

CARDIAC ACTION POTENTIAL

Membrane potential (membrane voltage or transmembrane potential) is the difference in electric potential between the interior and exterior of the cell, due to voltage changes across the cell membranes of heart cells.

SA node is a group of specialized cells, in the right atrium that generates action potential in the heart at a rate of 60 – 100 beats per minute.

Because of junctions that link the cardiomyocytes, action potential passes from one cell to other, causing atria and ventricles to contract. First atrial cells contract together followed by ventricular cells contraction. The ECG records this action potential activity of the heart.

Special types of voltage gated ions channels that are embedded in plasma membrane generate action potential.

During resting potential (negative) of cell, the channels are shut, and they will open again, if membrane reaches to threshold voltage.

As the channel opens, more inflow of sodium ions will take place, changing the electrochemical gradient. Further increasing membrane potential and eventually causing more channels to open, producing more electric current across the membrane. The process continues till all present ion channels are open, producing more electric current across the membrane. The process continues until all present ion channels are open. Until sodium channels are closed, no sodium ion can enter the cell. It is followed by activation of potassium channels causing an outward current of potassium ions, resulting in resting state.

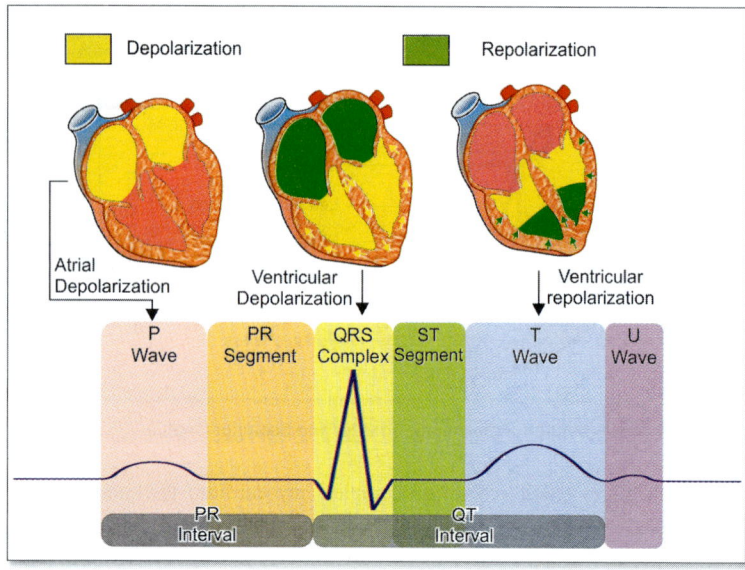

Fig. 1.5 ECG waveforms representing various phases of cardiac cycle

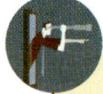

Note

Extended Plateau Phase

In cardiac action potential, there is an **extended plateau phase** (i.e., membrane remains at high voltage for few more milliseconds before being repolarized by potassium current). This extended plateau makes cardiac action potential differ from neuron action potential.

Phases of Cardiac Action Potential

There are **five phases** of cardiac action potential (Ventricle Myocyte) (Fig. 1.6 and Table 1.2).

- Phase 4
- Phase 0
- Phase 1
- Phase 2
- Phase 3

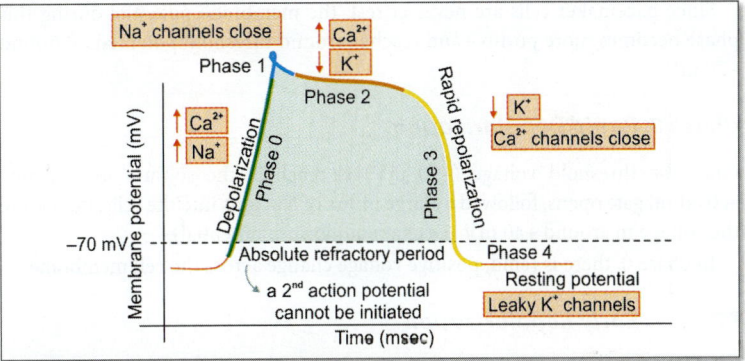

Fig. 1.6 Phases of cardiac action potential

Table 1.2 Cardiac action potential–summarized

Phases	Outcome	Mechanism
Phase 4	Resting phase	inside cell, K⁺ out; Cell membrane, Na⁺ ⊘
Phase 0	Rapid depolarization	Na⁺ in, Ca⁺⁺ in
Phase 1	Early repolarization	Na⁺ ⊘
Phase 2	Plateau Phase	Ca⁺⁺ in, K⁺ out
Phase 3	Rapid repolarization	Ca⁺⁺ ⊘, K⁺ out

Phase 4: Resting Phase

Resting membrane potential means that the ions that have flowed into the cell (i.e., Na^+ and Ca^{++}) and ions that have flowed out of the cell (i.e. K^+, Cl, HCO_3) are in perfect balance to each other.

The working myocardial cell has a resting membrane potential of approximately –90 mV.

During resting phase, the cardiomyocytes are at rest, in a period called **diastole**.

During this phase, the membrane is most permeable to K^+ ions; therefore resting membrane potential is determined by **potassium equilibrium potential.**

This phase is the interim between the end of rapid repolarization and start of next action potential.

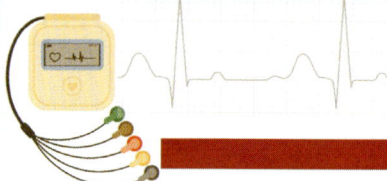

Since pacemaker cells are never at rest, the membrane potential during this phase becomes more positive and reaches around threshold potential of around –70 mV.

Phase 0: Rapid Depolarization

Once the threshold voltage (–70 mV) is reached, the sodium ion channel activation gate opens, followed by large influx of Na^+ ions into the cells, increasing the voltage to around +40 mV (i.e. Na^+ equilibrium potential).

In phase 0, there is rapid, positive voltage change across the cell membrane.

Phase 1: Early Repolarization

Na^+ channels close with rapid upstroke in membrane potential, thereby reducing Na^+ into the cells.

At the same time K^+ channels open, allowing K^+ ions to flow out of the cells, making membrane slightly more negative (+10 mV).

Phase 2: Plateau Phase

This phase is known as **plateau phase** because membrane potential remains constant. There is movement of Ca^{++} ions into the cell. This Ca binds and opens more Ca^{++} channels from sarcoplasmic reticulum within the cell allowing flow of calcium out of sarcoplasmic reticulum. This Ca^{++} causes contraction.

Phase 3: Rapid Repolarization

During this phase, calcium channel closes and repolarization starts, with outward movement of K^+ ions. The membrane voltage becomes increasingly negative and sodium channel inactivation is stopped. The sodium channel again can be excited.

There are two refractory periods in cardiac action potential.
- **Absolute refractory period (ARP)**
- **Relative refractory period (RRP)**

ARP is from phase 0 to part way through phase 3, during which it is impossible for the cardiac myocytes to produce another action potential. Second is **RRP**, that starts from end of phase 3 during which a stronger than usual stimulus is required to produce another action potential.

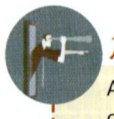

Note -

Anomalies or disturbances in cardiac action potential – congenital or injury (ischemic) can lead to arrhythmias.

Practice Questions

1. **Normal PR interval is:**
   a. 0.10-0.20 sec
   b. 0.11-0.21 sec
   c. 0.12-0.20 sec
   d. 0.10 – 0.21 sec

2. **Time period from initiation of atrial depolarization to initiation of ventricular depolarization is:**
   a. PR segment
   b. PR interval
   c. QT interval
   d. ST segment

3. **The cluster of cells with fastest rate of automaticity is:**
   a. SA node
   b. AV node
   c. Bundle branches
   d. Purkinje fibres

4. **The terms – "depolarization and repolarization" means respectively:**
   a. Relaxation and contraction respectively
   b. Contraction and relaxation respectively
   c. Both means contraction
   d. Both means relaxation

5. **In cardiac action potential phase 4 is:**
   a. Resting phase
   b. Depolarization phase
   c. Repolarization phase
   d. Plateau phase

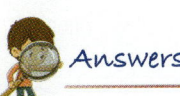 Answers

1. c   2. b   3. a   4. b   5. a

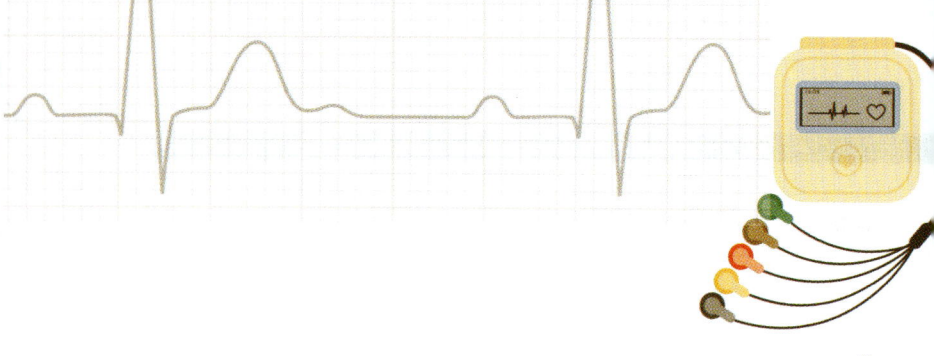

Electrocardiographic Leads

Chapter **2**

INTRODUCTION

- **Lead:** It is a connector to an electrode (Figs 2.1A and B) and is the one which traces the electrical potential difference between the two points (bipolar) or at one point (unipolar).
- **Electrode:** These are small gel pads which are conductive to electrical signals when, attached to the skin (Figs 2.1A and B).

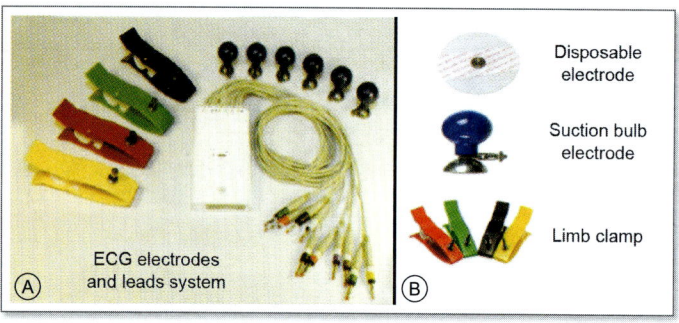

Disposable electrode

Suction bulb electrode

Limb clamp

ECG electrodes and leads system

(A)

(B)

Figs 2.1A and B A. ECG electrodes and lead system; B. Types of electrodes

In combination, electrocardiogram (ECG) leads are basically set of the electrodes having wires or cables, that are applied to one side to patient body surface and other end to the ECG machine.

Leads view the heart's electrical activity from the different angles and takes the different pictures of the same electrical stimulus from different angles or positions.

Let's imagine a toy house of a child with lots of windows. If you try to look inside the house from different windows, every time you will see the different perspective of inside, but the house remains same. Likewise in a heart, electrical stimulus is same, but it is captured by leads as cameras through different positions.

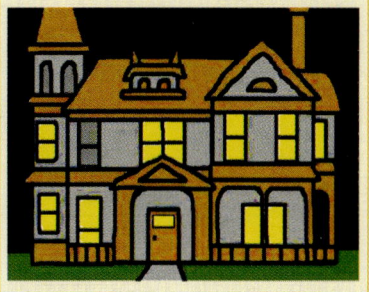

Standard ECG consists of 12 leads 6 limbs lead and 6 precordial leads (Fig. 2.2).

Standardized 12 leads ECG has, 10 leads placed on the body (limbs and chest). Because two leads share same electrode only 10 electrodes are required for the standardized 12 lead ECG. Each of this lead provides different view of electrical activity of the heart (Table 2.1).

Think about putting a different camera to focus on the different areas of the heart, and getting different images and then putting all the images together to get the idea what is going on in the heart.

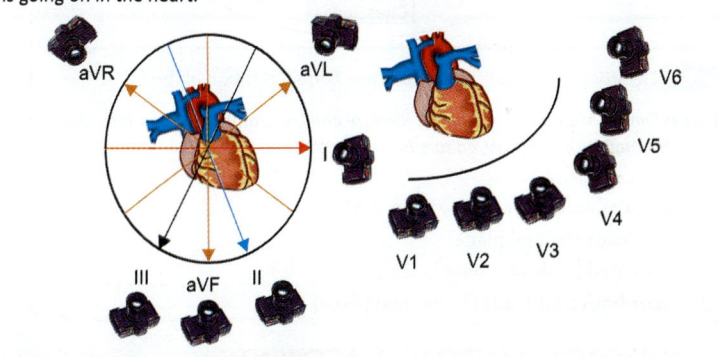

Fig. 2.2 12 Lead ECG system

12 ECG leads and area representing them

I Lateral	aVR	V1 Septal	V4 Anterior
II inferior	aVL Lateral	V2 Septal	V5 Septal
III Inferior	aVF Inferior	V3 Anterior	V6 Septal

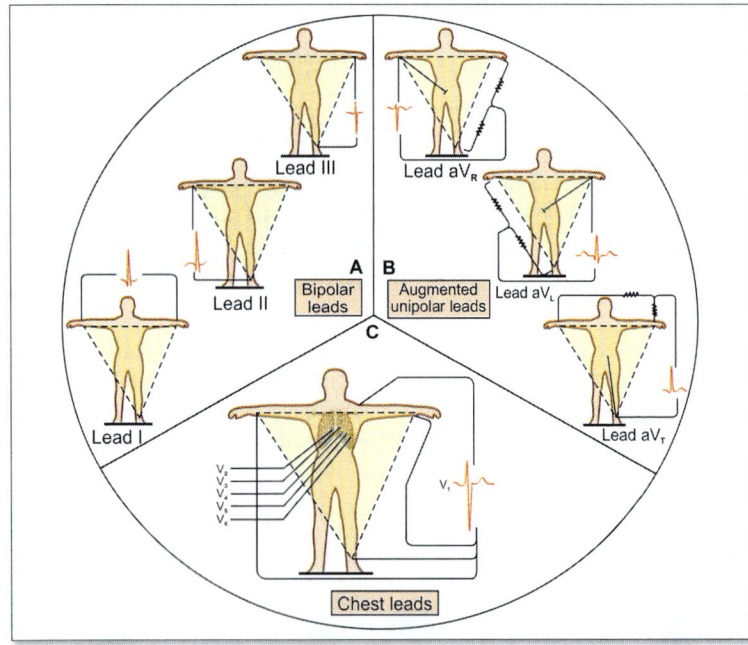

Chest leads

Fig. 2.3 Electrocardiographic leads with their correct position on body

(**Source:** *Clinical Methods: The History, Physical and Laboratory Examinations. 3rd edition. Walker HK, Hall WD, Hurst JW, editors.Boston: Butterworths; 1990*)

The leads are described as below (Fig. 2.3):
- **3 limbs leads** (frontal plane)
- **3 augmented leads** (frontal plane)
- **3 precordial/chest leads** (horizontal plane)

12 LEAD ECG ELECTRODE PLACEMENTS

Table 2.1 ECG leads placement

Leads			Electrode Placement
10 Leads	Chest leads	V1	4th Right ICS* at sternal border
		V2	4th Left ICS at sternal border
		V3	Mid/halfway between V2 and V4
		V4	5th ICS Midclavicular line (MCL)
		V5	5th ICS Anterior axillary line (AAL)
		V6	5th ICS Midaxillary line (MAL)

Contd...

Leads			Electrode Placement
	Limb leads	aVR	Right arm
		aVL	Left arm
		aVF	left foot
		N	Right foot
Abbreviations: ICS, Intercostal Space; aVR, augmented vector right arm; aVL, augmented vector left arm; aVF, augmented vector foot (left).			

Precordial Leads (Chest Leads) (Figs 2.4 and 2.5)

Designated as capital letter "**V**" and numbering given as 1, 2, 3, 4, 5, 6 there are total six **precordial Leads** which are also called as chest leads. These leads view the heart electrical activity from the horizontal plane. These are unipolar leads, with electrodes placed on the chest as positive pole with single zero reference point for all precordial leads (Fig. 2.4).

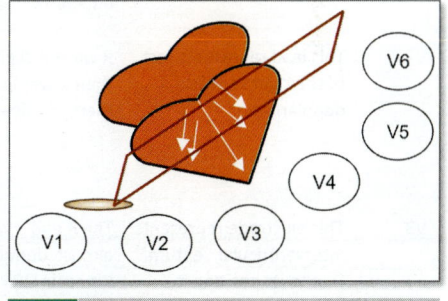

Fig. 2.4 Precordial leads

To understand it more clearly have a look on a normal ECG - precordial leads V1, V2, V3, V4, V5, V6 given in Figure 2.5.

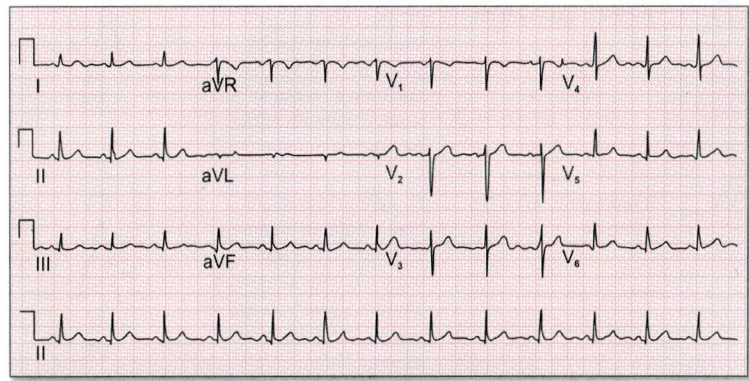

Fig. 2.5 Normal ECG – Checkout precordial leads V1 to V6 to understand QRS normal morphology in precordial leads refer Table 2.2

Table 2.2 shows and explains the morphology in the chest leads. For their placement *see* Figure 2.6.

Table 2.2 Chest leads and QRS morphology

Chest Leads	Description	QRS Morphology	
V1	It represents electrical potential in atria, septum and part of right ventricle.	There is a small R wave formed because of septum depolarization, deep S wave by subsequent ventricle depolarization activation	r / S / V1
V2	This lead represents rest of the right ventricle depolarization.	R wave is slightly bigger than it was in V1 and there is a deep S wave	R / S / V2
V3	This electrode represents interventricular septum. Due to its position it is the transitional lead between left and right ventricle potentials.	The R and S waves are almost identical called **Biphasic QRS**	R / S / V3
V4	It represents left ventricle apex potential.	Because ventricle wall at apex region is most thickest, therefore in this lead there will be tall R wave and small **S wave** (right ventricle depolarization)	R / S / V4
V5	It represents left ventricle	Compared to apex region walls are thinner therefore in this lead R wave is not as tall as in V4. There is a **small q wave** representing septum depolarization	R / q / V5

Contd...

Chest Leads	Description	QRS Morphology	
V6	It represents left ventricle	R wave is not as tall as in V4. There is a small Q wave.	R q V6

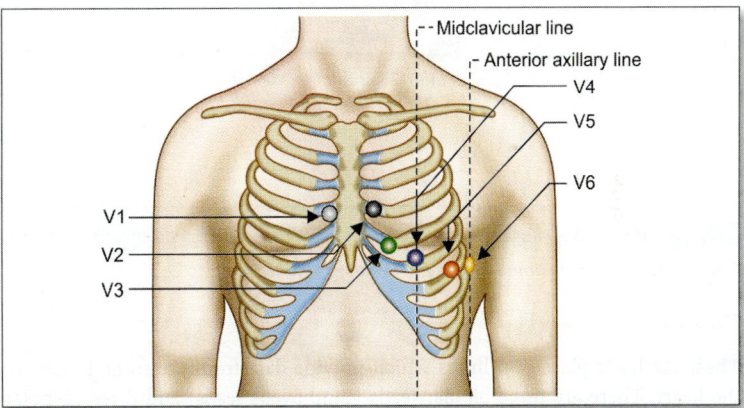

		Transitional zone	R V4	R V5	R V6
r V1 S	R V2 S	R V3 S	s	q	q

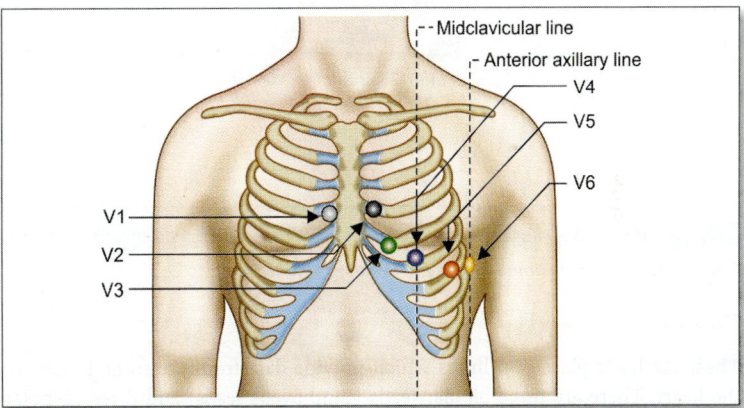

Fig. 2.6 Precordial lead placement

Augmented Limb Leads

Augmented limb leads (aVR, aVL, aVF) are unipolar leads and take one limb electrodes as positive pole and take average of input from other two leads as a negative point or zero reference points (Table 2.3 and Fig. 2.7).

Table 2.3 Details of augmented limb leads

Augmented limb leads	aVR	aVL	AVF
Positive pole	Right arm (RA)	Left arm (LA)	Left foot/leg (LL)
Negative/zero reference point	Average of LA and LL	Average of RA and LL	Average of RA and LA
Figures Illustrating augmented leads			

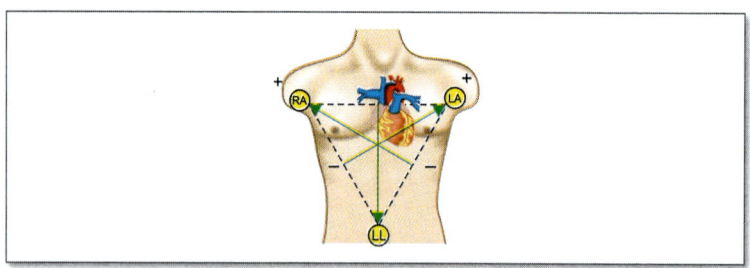

Fig. 2.7 Augmented limb leads placements

Abbreviations: *RA, Right arm; LA, Left arm; LL, Lower limb/left leg*

Bipolar Limb leads

These are leads placed on limbs which provide data from the frontal plane of the heart. There are three bipolar leads (Einthoven's leads) and three unipolar augmented leads.

Lead I, II and III are considered as bipolar leads since they measure the electrical potential between the two of the three limb leads (aVR, aVL and aVF). Depending on position angle from where electrical activity of the heart is viewed, the point of view is considered as positive terminal and the starting point is considered as negative terminal or zero reference (Table 2.4).

Table 2.4 Details of bipolar limb leads

Bipolar Leads	Lead I	Lead II	Lead III
Represents electrical potential difference between	RA (−) to LA (+)	RA (−) to LL (+)	LA (−) to LL (+)
Looking for heart electrical activity from	Left side	Inferior left	Inferior right
Figures Illustrating bipolar leads			

EINTHOVEN'S TRIANGLE

Theorized by "Willem Einthoven". In electrocardiography, the three imaginary limb leads are formed, as an inverted equilateral triangle called Einthoven's Triangle. The three bipolar leads together form an Einthoven's triangle (Fig. 2.8).

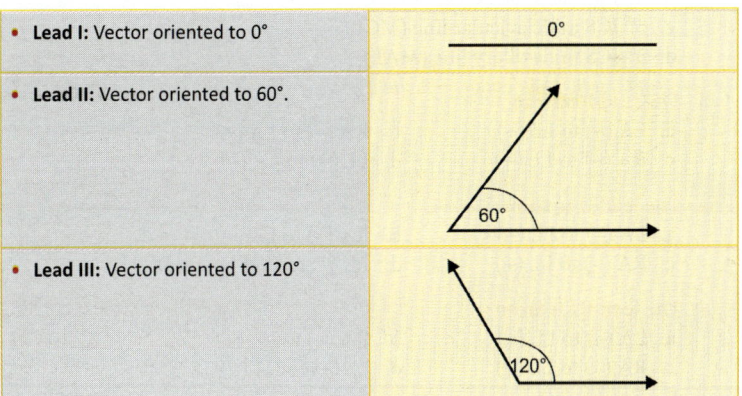

• **Lead I:** Vector oriented to 0°	0°
• **Lead II:** Vector oriented to 60°.	60°
• **Lead III:** Vector oriented to 120°	120°

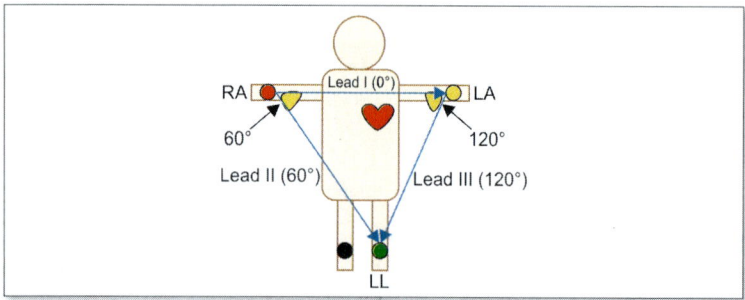

RA

Fig. 2.8 Three bipolar leads placement forming einthoven's triangle

Abbreviations: *RA, Right arm; LA, Left arm; LL, Lower limb/left leg*

 Practice Questions

1. **In a 12 lead ECG, how many electrodes are attached:**
   a. 12
   b. 11
   c. 10
   d. 9

2. **The placement of precodial lead – V4 is**
   a. 5th ICS anterior axillary line (AAL)
   b. 4th right ICS* at sternal border
   c. 5th ICS midclavicular line (MCL)
   d. 5th ICS midaxillary line (MAL)

3. **The lead I is from**
   a. LA (–) to LL (+)
   b. RA (–) to LA (+)
   c. RA (–) to LL (+)
   d. LL (+) to LA (–)

4. **The lead II is from**
   a. LA (–) to LL (+)
   b. RA (–) to LA (+)
   c. RA (–) to LL (+)
   d. LL (+) to LA (–)

5. **The lead III is from**
   a. LA (–) to LL (+)
   b. RA (–) to LA (+)
   c. RA (–) to LL (+)
   d. LL (+) to LA (–)

 Answers

1. c   2. c   3. b   4. c   5. a

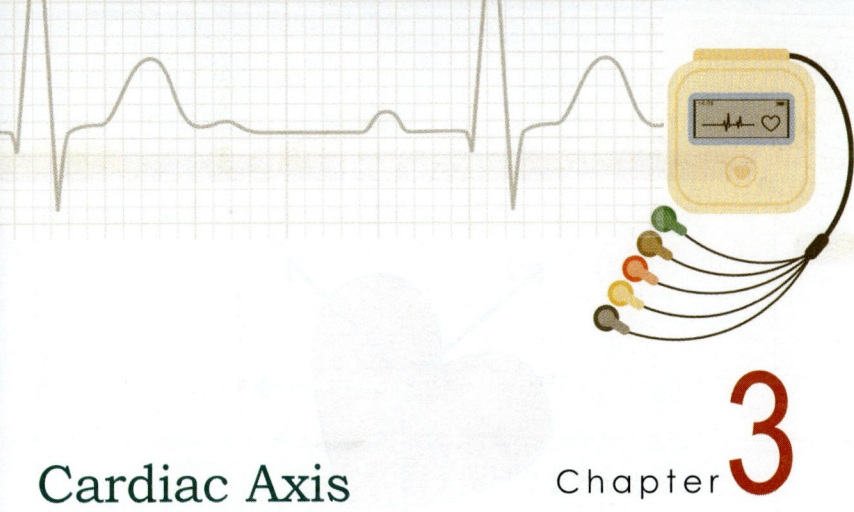

Cardiac Axis

Chapter 3

INTRODUCTION

At a given time, with the same electrical stimulus, different vectors are generated in the heart in different directions. Of these different vectors in different direction, there is an average vector, which gives cardiac axis. The largest and longest vector is the net vector (Fig. 3.1). The length of the vector indicates its magnitude.

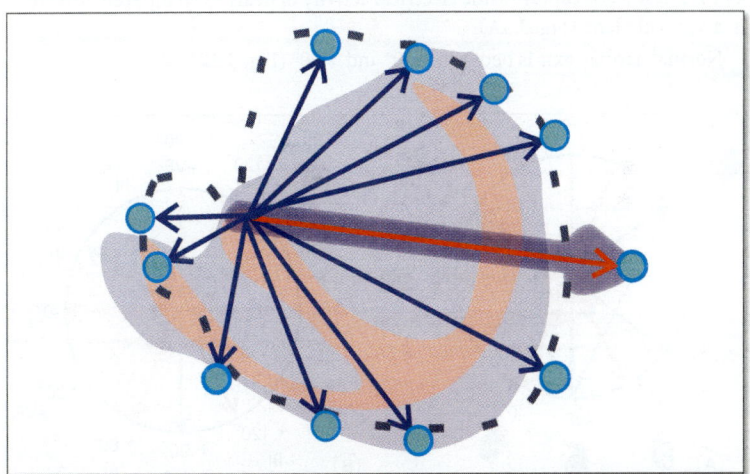

Fig. 3.1 Net electrical vector (red arrow)

The net or average direction of the electrical potential during the depolarization is the **cardiac axis**. The vector generated by the electrical stimulation has a magnitude, direction as well as polarity and is measurable. The net movement of the vector is downward and leftward (Fig. 3.2).

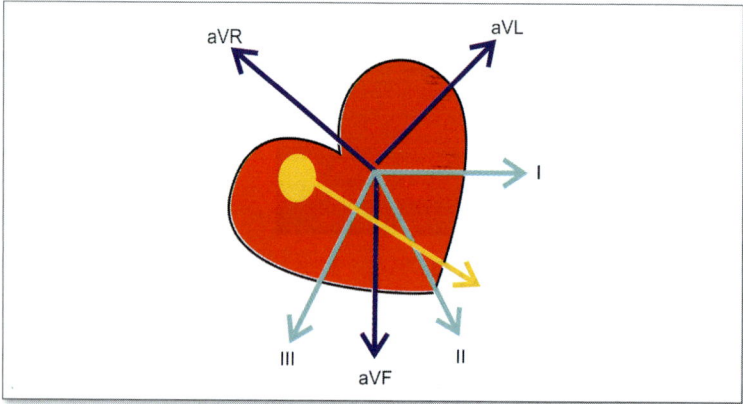

Fig. 3.2 Net cardiac electromotive vector direction - downward and leftward (yellow arrow)

The cardiac axis is determined by 6 bipolar leads (lead I, II, III, aVR, aVL and aVF). These leads capture same electrical activity of heart from different direction in a vertical plane (Fig. 3.3A).

Normal cardiac axis is between – 30° and + 90° (Fig. 3.3B).

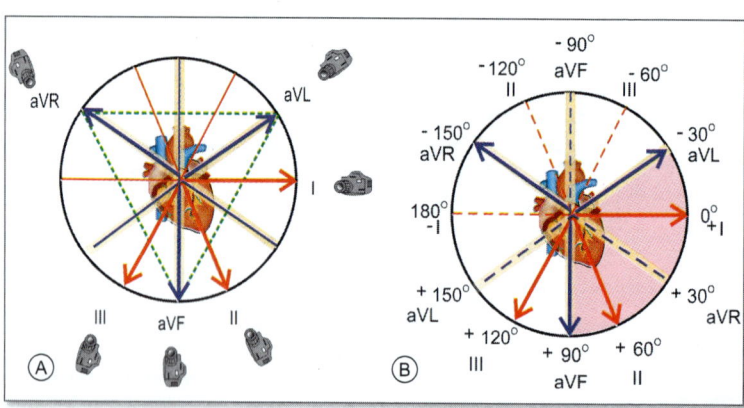

Figs 3.3A and B Bipolar leads and normal cardiac axis

The cardiac axis is determined by the **Hexa-axial reference system (HRS)** which is derived from the Einthoven's Triangle (Table 3.1).

Table 3.1 Hexaaxial reference system (HRS)

Leads	Positive Pole	Negative Pole
I	0°	+/−180°
aVF	+90°	−90°
II	+60°	−120°
III	+120°	−60°
aVR	−150°	+30°
aVL	−30°	+150°

Note -

The direction of movement of vector is the positive pole shown by arrow and direction away from the movement of vector is the negative pole

DEVIATION IN CARDIAC AXIS

The normal cardiac axis is downward and leftward, but this net movement of vector can be deviated in certain conditions and may cause axis deviation – right axis deviation, left axis deviation, or may be extreme axis deviation (Fig. 3.4). The deviations in cardiac axis have been summarized in Table 3.2.

Table 3.2 Deviation in cardiac axis

Axis	Angle	Diagramatic Illustration
Normal cardiac axis	-30° and 90°	- 90° - 30° - 180° 180° 90° Normal axis

Contd...

Axis	Angle	Diagramatic Illustration
Left axis deviation	-30° and -90°	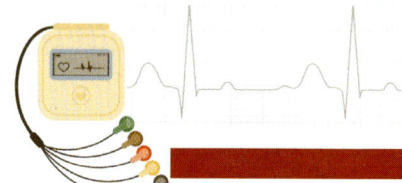Left axis deviation
Right axis deviation	90° and 180°	Right axis deviation
Extreme axis deviation	-90° and -180°	Extreme axis deviation

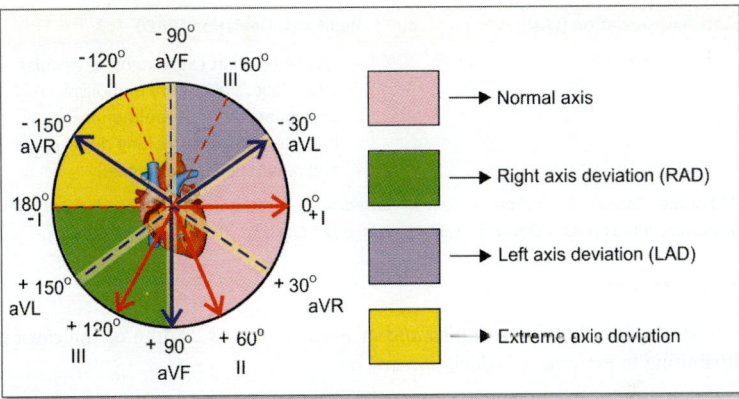

Fig. 3.4 Cardiac axis deviation

Causes of Axis Deviation

The causes of axis deviations have been given in Table 3.3.

Table 3.3 Causes of axis deviation**

Left Axis Deviation (LAD)	Right Axis Deviation (RAD)
• Normal variation (physiologic, often age-related change) • Left ventricular hypertrophy • Conduction defects: left bundle branch block, left anterior fascicular block • Inferior wall myocardial infarction • Preexcitation syndromes (e.g., Wolff-Parkinson-White syndrome) • Ventricular ectopic rhythms (e.g., ventricular tachycardia) • Congenital heart disease (e.g., primum atrial septal defect, endocardial cushion defect) • Hyperkalaemia • Emphysema • Mechanical shift, such as with expiration or raised diaphragm (e.g., pregnancy, ascites, abdominal tumor, organomegaly) • Pacemaker-generated rhythm or paced rhythm	• Normal variation (e.g., children, young adults) • Limb-lead reversal (left-arm and right-arm electrodes) • Right ventricular overload syndromes (acute or chronic) • Right ventricular hypertrophy • Conduction defects: left posterior fascicular block, right bundle branch block • Lateral wall myocardial infarction • Preexcitation syndromes (e.g., Wolff-Parkinson-White syndrome) • Ventricular ectopic rhythms (e.g., ventricular tachycardia) • Congenital heart disease (e.g., secundum atrial septal defect) • Dextrocardia • Left pneumothorax • Mechanical shift, such as with inspiration or emphysema

Contd...

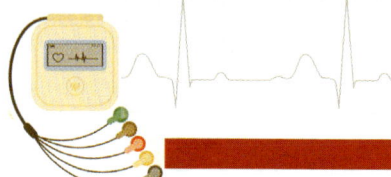
Left Axis Deviation (LAD)	Right Axis Deviation (RAD)
	• Conditions that cause right-ventricular strain (e.g., pulmonary embolism, pulmonary stenosis, pulmonary hypertension, chronic lung disease, and resultant cor pulmonale)

(**Source:** *Kashou A, Kashou H, Kent K, Rebedew D. Electrical Axis (Normal, Right Axis Deviation, and Left Axis Deviation). Statpearls. 2018 Oct 27*).

Extreme Axis Deviation

It is also referred as "*No Man's Land or north west axis*". Some of the causes attributing to extreme axis deviation are:

- Emphysema
- Hyperkalaemia
- Ventricular tachycardia
- Artificial pacemaker rhythms, etc.

This deviation frequently is present in ventricular tachycardia and artificial pacemaker rhythms. It may be seen in emphysema and hyperkalaemia and can indicate lead transposition.

DETERMINING CARDIAC AXIS

When an electric stimulus travels towards the direction of the lead or positive pole, positive deflection occurs and when the electrical stimulus travels away from the lead, negative deflection occurs (Figs 3.5A and B). If electrical stimulus moves 90° to the lead, then there will be equal positive and negative deflection, called **equiphasic deflection** (Fig. 3.6).

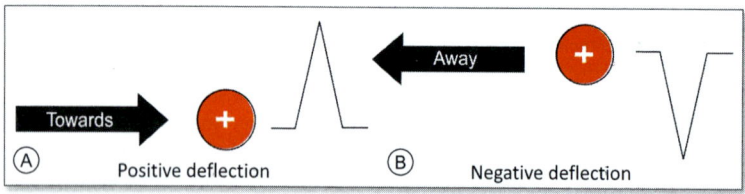

Figs 3.5A and B (A) Positive deflection; (B) Negative deflection

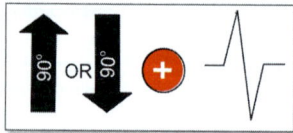

Fig. 3.6 Isoelectric or equiphasic deflection

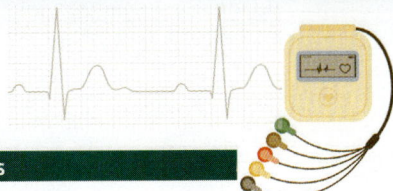

Isoelectric Lead Method

- This method consists of finding the lead with iso-electric (equiphasic) deflection.
- Once the isoelectric lead is identified, it is consider that axis line will be perpendicular to this isoelectric lead.
- Look for the lead which is nearest to the axis line.
- If the QRS complex is positive in this lead, (which is nearest to the axis line direction) then the axis direction is towards the same direction as that of the lead.
- If the QRS complex is negative in the nearest lead it means that axis direction is opposite.
- Example of isoelectric method in a normal ECG has been shown in Figure 3.7.

Let's learn with an example

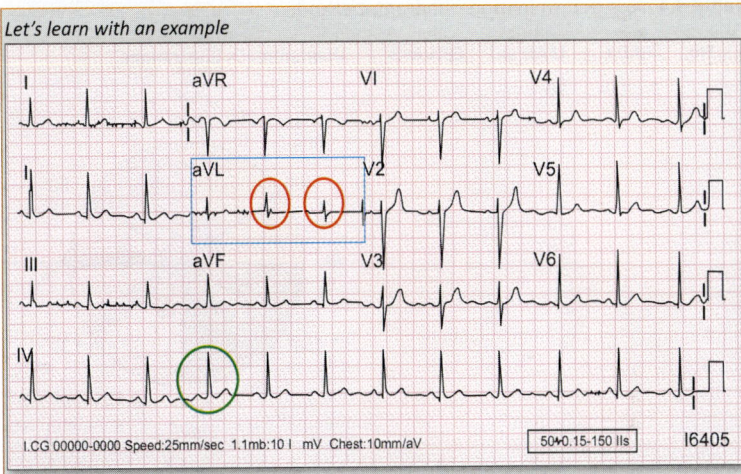

I   aVR   VI   V4
II   aVL   V2   V5
III aVF   V3   V6
IV

I.CG 00000-0000 Speed:25mm/sec 1.1mb:10 I mV Chest:10mm/aV   50*0.15-150 IIs   I6405

Fig. 3.7 Normal ECG

Example - Axis determination by Isoelectric Method

1.	Identify isoelectric lead	AvL lead is isoelectric	
2.	Look for nearest lead to perpendicular axis direction (yellow line)	Lead II is the nearest lead	

Contd...

3.	Look for deflection in the nearest lead	Lead II has positive deflection	
4.	Interpretation		Axis direction is towards lead II, confirming that axis is near about 600 and within normal limit

Quadrant Method

This method consists of looking for QRS deflection in lead I and lead aVF (Table 3.4).

Table 3.4 Axis determination-quadrant method

S. No.	LEAD I	LEAD aVF	QRS Axis	Diagrammatic illustrations
1.	Positive	Positive	Normal axis	
2.	Negative	Positive	Right Axis deviation (RAD)	

Contd...

S. No.	LEAD I	LEAD aVF	QRS Axis	Diagrammatic illustrations
3.	Positive	Negative	Left Axis Deviation (LAD)	
4.	Negative	Negative	Extreme Axis Deviation	

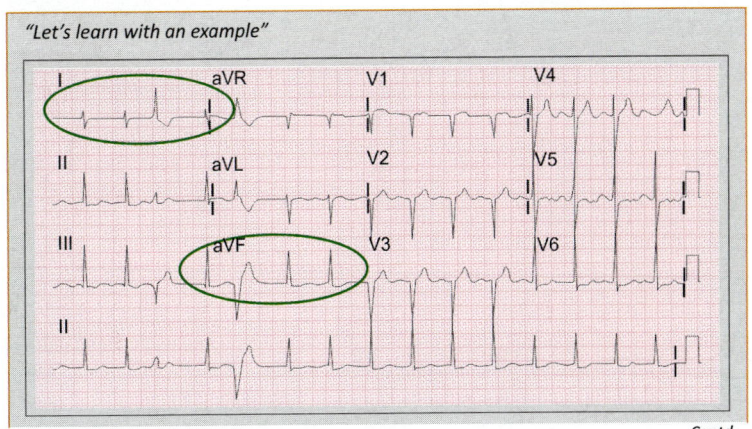

"Let's learn with an example"

Contd...

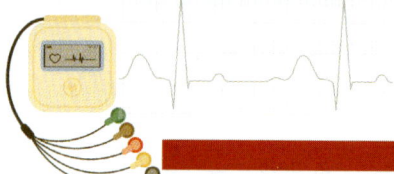
Step 1: Identify lead I deflection–negative
Step 2: Identify lead aVF deflection–positive
Step 3: Imagine or draw.

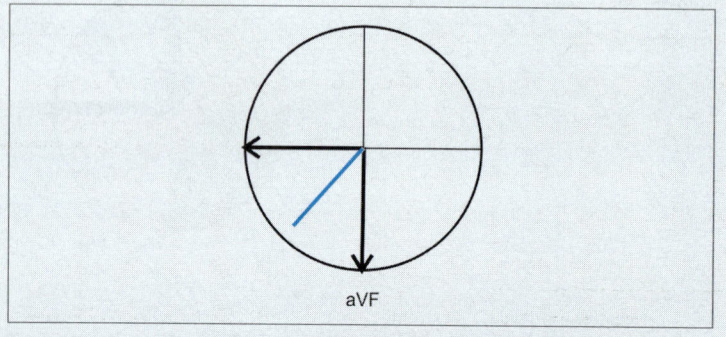

Step 4: Lead I is negative and lead aVF is positive, it is **right axis deviation**.

Accurate Axis Determination Method

In this method lead I and lead aVF, QRS amplitude is measured in mm, and plotted together to find the accurate axis.

To calculate net amplitude of QRS, substract Q or S wave amplitude from R wave amplitude. Value can be negative or positive (if negative use minus sign).

For example, if S wave magnitude is 8 mm, R wave magnitude is 6 mm. The QRS amplitude for this will be –2 mm.

"Let's learn with an example"

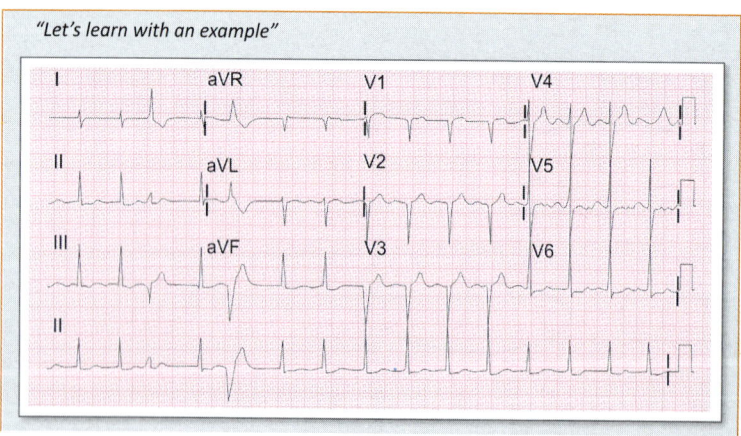

Contd...

Step 1: Lead I R wave amplitude = 2 mm

Step 2: Lead I S wave amplitude = –3 mm

Step 3: Net QRS wave amplitude = –1 mm

Step 4: Lead aVF R wave amplitude = 12 mm

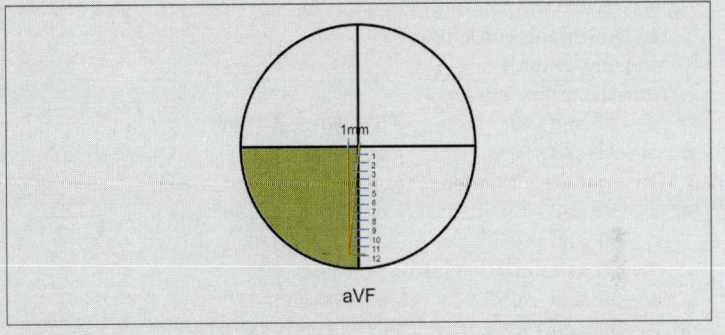

Step 5: Plot the amplitude to find the net deflection-**right axis deviation**

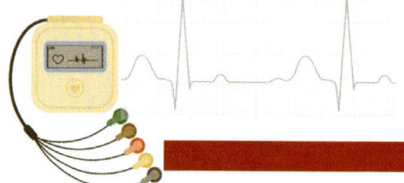

  Practice Questions

1. **The net movement of cardiac vector is towards**
   a. Downward and rights ward
   b. Upward and left ward
   c. Downwards and leftward
   d. Only upwards

2. **Normal cardiac axis is:**
   a. −30° and −90°   b. −90° and −180°
   c. −30° and +90°   d. 90° and 180°

3. **The right axis deviation is from -**
   a. −30° and −90°   b. −90° and −180°
   c. −30° and +90°   d. 90° and 180°

4. **The left axis deviation is from**
   a. −30° and −90°   b. −90° and −180°
   c. −30° and +90°   d. 90° and 180°

5. **Identify axis deviation in given ECG**

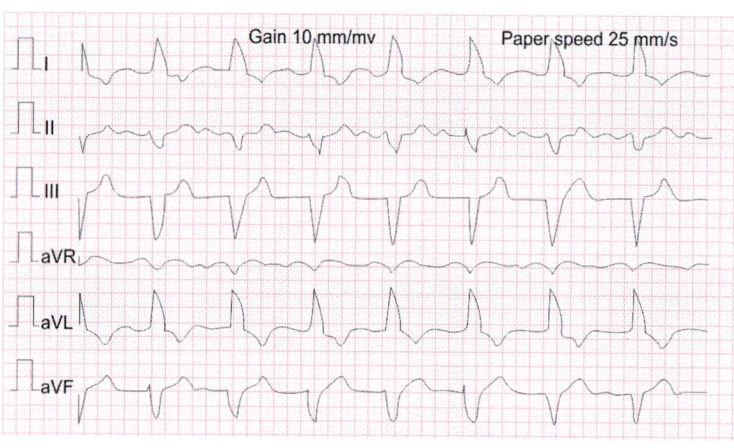

   a. Normal axis deviation   b. Right axis deviation
   c. Left axis deviation   d. Extreme axis deviation

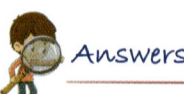 Answers

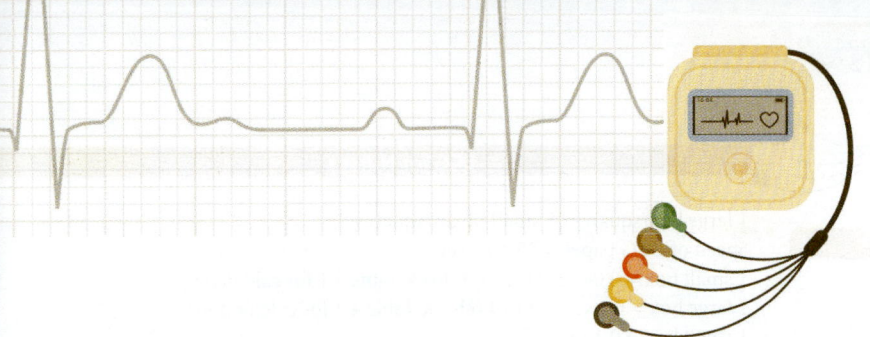

ECG Paper and Waveforms

Chapter 4

INTRODUCTION

Electrocardiogram (ECG) paper is a strip of graph paper with large and small grids. On horizontal axis there is time in seconds and on vertical axis there is the voltage in mV.

Standard calibration of ECG machine is in a way that 1 mill volt (mV) produces a 10 mm of deflection vertically and 5 milli meter (mm) of width horizontally (Fig. 4.1).

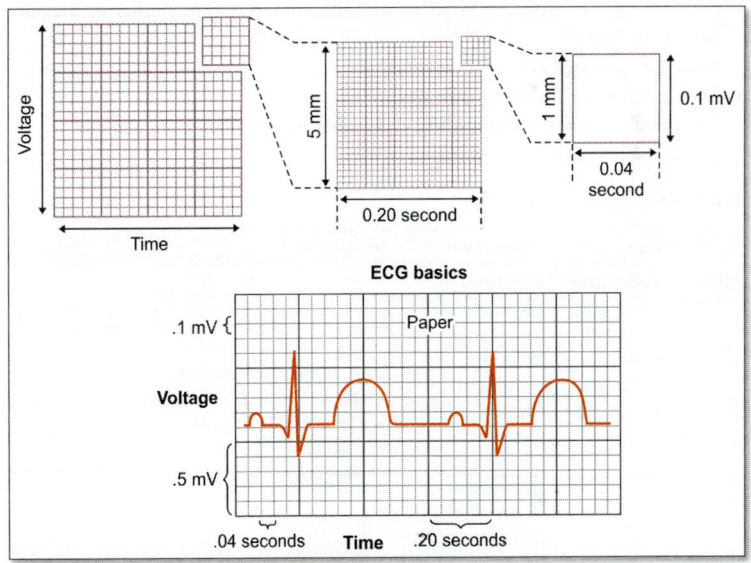

Fig. 4.1 ECG Grid

(**Source:** *Becker DE. Fundamentals of electrocardiography interpretation. Anesthesia progress. 2006 Jun;53(2):53-64.*)

1 large box/square = 5 small boxes/squares
Speed of ECG paper = 25 mm/sec
1 small box = 0.04 sec (1 mm) (check Table 4.1 for calculation)
1 large box = 0.2 sec (5 mm) (check Table 4.1 for calculation)
1 small box = 0.1 mV
1 large box = 0.5 mV

Table 4.1 ECG paper calculation

Question	Calculation	Answer
If 25 mm is covered in 1 sec, then 1 mm completes in how many seconds?	25 mm = 1 sec 1 mm = x sec	x sec = 1 × 1/25 = **0.04 sec** **Therefore, 1 mm** **(1 small box) is of 0.04 sec**
1 small box is of 0.04 sec, then 1 big box is of how many seconds?	1 small box or 1 mm = 0.04 sec 1 big box = 5 mm	1 big box = 5 × 0.04 = **0.2 sec** **Therefore, 1 big box is of 0.2 sec**

ANALYSIS OF ECG

The steps to analyze the ECG are as follows (Table 4.2):
- Determine whether rhythm is regular or irregular.
- Look for P wave. Are all P waves similar?
- Look for QRS complexes. Whether all QRS complexes are similar or they are narrow or broad?
- Are all PR interval are same or varying?
- Look for T wave and its morphology.
- Look that all waves are preceding each other in a normal sequence
- Is the rate normal?

Table 4.2 Steps of ECG Analysis

	Steps	Description	Images
Step 1	Determine whether rhythm is regular or irregular?	Regularity of the rhythm determines atrial and ventricular rhythm. The interval between QRS complexes (R – R intervals) and between P waves (P – P intervals), should be consistent.	R R Look at the R-R distances • Regular (equidistant apart) • Occasionally irregular • Regularly irregular • Irregularly irregular

Contd...

	Steps	Description	Images
Step 2	Assess P wave. Are all P waves are similar?	P wave – **<0.12 sec** P waves denotes atrial depolarization	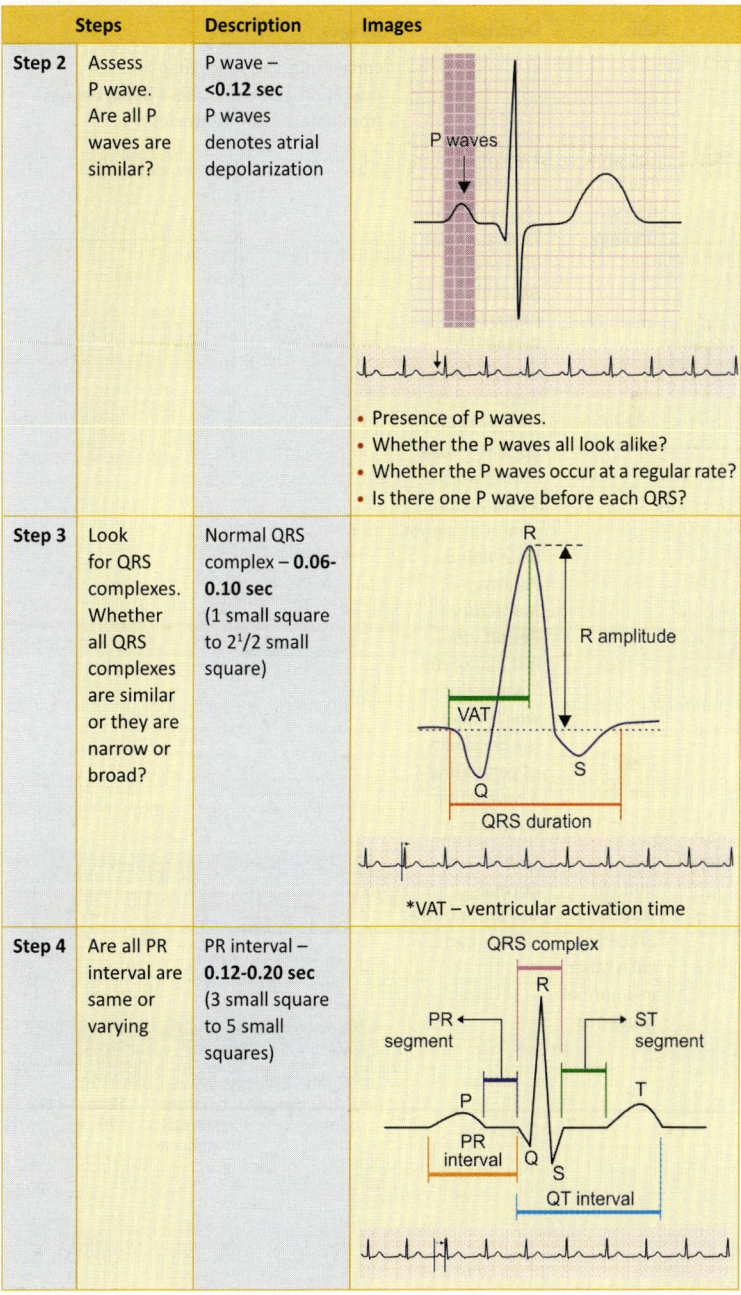 • Presence of P waves. • Whether the P waves all look alike? • Whether the P waves occur at a regular rate? • Is there one P wave before each QRS?
Step 3	Look for QRS complexes. Whether all QRS complexes are similar or they are narrow or broad?	Normal QRS complex – **0.06-0.10 sec** (1 small square to 2$\frac{1}{2}$ small square)	*VAT – ventricular activation time
Step 4	Are all PR interval are same or varying	PR interval – **0.12-0.20 sec** (3 small square to 5 small squares)	

Contd...

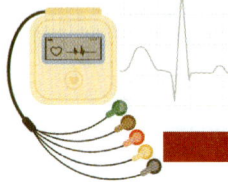

Steps		Description	Images
			Longer intervals more than >0.20 sec indicate that the impulse is being delayed from entering the ventricles
Step 5	Look for T wave and its morphology	T wave denotes ventricular repolarization T wave = 0.10-0.25 sec **Absolute Refractory Period** – interval from beginning of QRS complex to apex of T wave during which a new action potential cannot be initiated. **Relative Refractory Period** –the last half of the T wave, during which there is a possibility of generating a new action potential.	T waves
Step 6	Look that all waves are preceding each other in a normal sequence	This assures normal sequence of the cardiac cycle.	Normal sinus rhythm

Heart rate	Rhythm	P wave	PR interval (in seconds)	QRS (in seconds)
60–100 bpm	Regular	Before each QRS, identical	.12 to .20	<.12

Contd...

	Steps	Description	Images
Step 7	Is the rate normal	Normal HR (adults) = 60 – 100 bpm Sinus bradycardia = <60 bpm Sinus tachycardia = >100 bpm	The heart rate is to be calculated using rule of 1500 or rule of 300 (mentioned in chapter)
Step 8	Any ectopic beat?	Ectopic beats are those that arise earlier than the next normal beat.	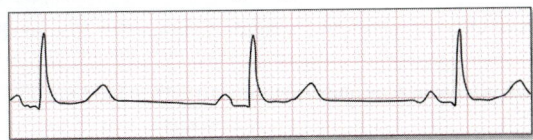

DETERMINING HEART RATE

When Heart Rate is Regular

Rule of 300

Count the number of large boxes between two R-R intervals (ventricular rate) or two P – P interval and divide 300 by the counted number.

(Reason: It is divided by 300, because heart rate is calculated in beats per minute (60 seconds)

Therefore $300 \times 0.20 = 60$ seconds)

Example 1 Calculate the HR from figure given below:

Solution: R – R interval = 6 big squares

Heart rate = 300/ No. of big boxes = 300/6 = 50 bpm (Bradycardia)

Rule of 1500

Count the number of small boxes between two R-R intervals (ventricular rate) or two P – P intervals (atrial rate) and divide the counted number by 1500.

(**Reason:** It is divided by 1500 because heart rate is calculated in beats per minute (60 seconds)

Therefore $1500 \times 0.04 = 60$ seconds

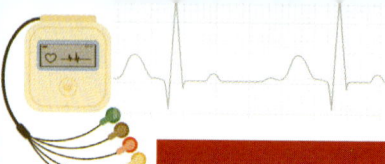

Example 2: Calculate the HR from ECG.

Solution: R – R interval = 30 small boxes

Heart rate = 1500/ No. of small boxes = 1500/30 = 50 bpm (Bradycardia)

When Heart Rate is Irregular

When HR is irregular, the rule of 300 or 1500 will not be an accurate method because QRS varies in irregular rhythms.

In irregular rhythms, number of QRS complexes are counted in 3 seconds or 6 seconds strip [(mostly 3 seconds interval are marked on ECG paper) and multiplied by 20 or 10 respectively].

1 big box = 0.20 sec

How many boxes (y) = 3 sec

Y = 3/0.20 = 15 big boxes

3 second strip = 15 big boxes

6 second strip = 30 big boxes

Example 3: Calculate the HR from ECG from figure given below:

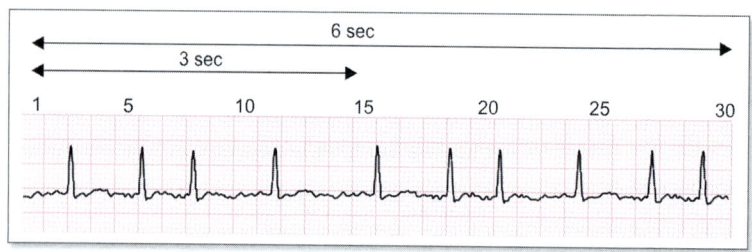

Solution: No. of QRS complexes in 3 seconds rhythm = 5 × 20 = 100 bpm

Or

No. of QRS complexes in 6 seconds rhythm = 10 × 10 = 100 bpm

Example 4: Calculate the HR from ECG from figure given below:

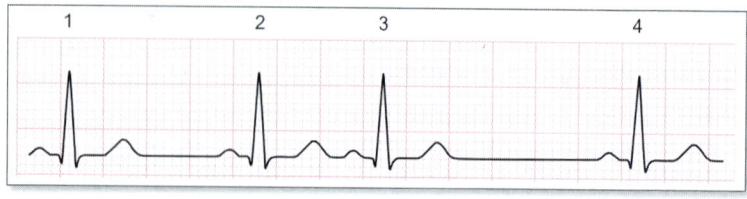

Solution: This is a 3 seconds rhythm (15 big boxes)
No. of QRS complexes in 3 seconds rhythm = 4 × 20 = 80 bpm

ECG WAVEFORMS

P wave

P wave represents atrial depolarization. Characteristics of P wave have been described in Table 4.3.

Table 4.3 Characteristics of P wave

Characteristics	• First positive deflection, assessment of ECG starts with P wave • Small, positive, smooth, upright wave – one preceding each QRS complex • With sinus rhythm, P wave is always positive in Lead II • In lead V1, p wave is occasionally biphasic, with negative deflection less than 1 mm • Amplitude of p wave is less than 2.5 mm	
Duration	≤ 0.12 sec	
Abnormality	With abnormal P wave, there will be change in the wave contour **P – Mitrale** **Cause –** left atrial enlargement, mostly in mitral stenosis. **Appearance –** second hump in the p wave in lead II, and there may be enhanced negative deflection of p wave in V1 lead (wide notched P waves)	II V₁
	P – Pulmonale **Cause –** right atrial enlargement, may be due to pulmonic valve stenosis or increased resistance to pulmonary circulation **Appearance –** Increased amplitude of p wave in lead II, V1 (tall peaked P waves)	II
	Others • Saw tooth shape p wave in atrial flutter • No p waves or fibrillatory p wave in atrial fibrillation	
Management	Treatment of underlying diseases condition	

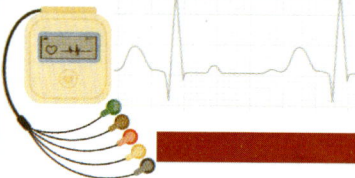
Nursing Management	Assess patient for atrial arrhythmias like atrial fibrillation, atrial flutter Patient in atrial fibrillation are mostly on anticoagulant therapy to prevent any CVA. It is the responsibility of the health professional to teach patient about importance of anticoagulation therapy, foods to be modified to have an effective anticoagulation and significance of regular PT/INR.

QRS Wave

QRS wave represents ventricular depolarization.

There are three waves in QRS complex – Q, R and S wave

The first wave Q is negative deflection, then first positive wave is R wave and next negative deflection is S wave.

If in a QRS complex all waves are large, it is denoted by capital letters (QRS) and if all waves are small then it is debnoted by small regular letters (qrs). There can be different patterns of a QRS complex (Tables 4.4 and 4.5).

Table 4.4 Characteristics of QRS waves

Characteristics	• Q wave is first negative deflection from baseline, following p wave • R wave is first positive deflection following Q wave. Since R wave depolarizes maximum ventricle mass, it is largest of 3 waves in a complex. • S wave is first negative deflection following R wave. • QRS is completely negative in aVR and maximum positive in lead II • R wave should be <26 mm in V5-V6 • R wave amplitude in V5/V6 + S wave in V1, should not be more than <35 mm
Duration	0.06-0.10 sec not exceeding <0.12 sec
Abnormality	Abnormality in QRS complex can be caused by variety of causes. Common causes are: • Left ventricular hypertrophy • Right ventricular hypertrophy • Bundle branch blocks (discussed in chapter 10) • Axis deviation (discussed in chapter 3)
	Left Ventricular Hypertrophy (LVH) **Cause** – May be caused by mitral valve disease, aortic valve disease, or systemic hypertension. **Appearance** - Tall S-wave is seen in precordial leads V_1 and V_2 and a tall R-wave in leads V_5 and V_6 (>35 mm) **Sokolow –lyon criteria** $\boxed{(R_{V5} \text{ or } R_{V6}) + (S_{V1} \text{ or } S_{V2}) > 35 \text{ min}}$ R wave in V5/V6 + S wave amplitude in V1/V2 = >35 mm = indicates LVH

Contd...

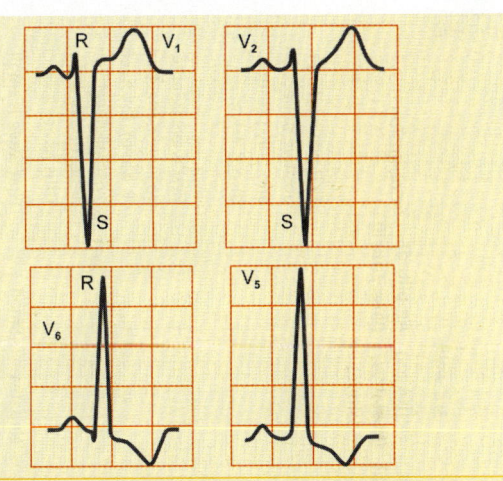

Right Ventricular Hypertrophy RVH

Cause – May be caused by right ventricle overload due to pulmonary valve stenosis, tricuspid insufficiency, or pulmonary hypertension etc.

Appearance – Large R wave i.e. increased amplitude in lead V1 and V2

Wide S wave in lead V1 and V2

Wide r wave in lead V5 and V6

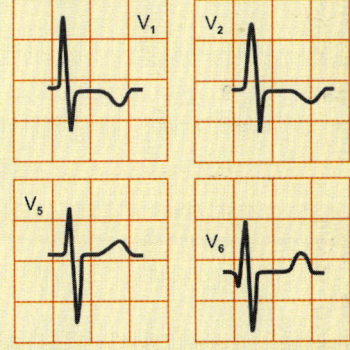

Management	Treatment of underlying disease condition
Nursing Management	Educate patient regarding underlying disease condition and importance of adherence to medical treatment

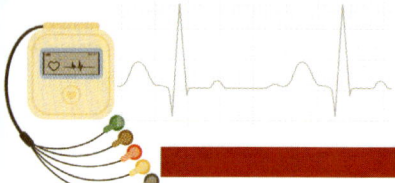

TABLE 4.5 Comparative analysis of QRS wave patterns

QRS Waveform Types	1st wave			2nd wave			3rd wave			Conclusion
	Present (yes/no)	Deflection (negative/ positive)	Amplitude (large/ small)	Present (yes/no)	Deflection (negative/ positive)	Amplitude (large/ small)	Present (yes/no)	Deflection (negative/ positive)	Amplitude (large/small)	
R	Yes	Positive	Large	No	–	–	No	–	–	First wave is large positive deflection and only present thus R wave
Rs	Yes	Positive	Large	Yes	Negative	Small	No	–	–	First wave is large positive deflection (R wave), followed by small negative deflection (s wave) Thus Rs
qRs	Yes	Negative	Small	Yes	Positive	Large	Yes	Negative	Small	First wave is small negative deflection (q wave), followed by large positive deflection (R wave), followed by small negative deflection (s wave) Thus qRs

Contd...

QRS Waveform Types	1st wave			2nd wave			3rd wave			Conclusion
	Present (yes/no)	Deflection (negative/ positive)	Amplitude (large/ small)	Present (yes/no)	Deflection (negative/ positive)	Amplitude (large/ small)	Present (yes/no)	Deflection (negative/ positive)	Amplitude (large/small)	
QR	Yes	Negative	Large	Yes	Positive	Large	No	–	–	First wave is large negative deflection (Q wave), followed by large negative deflection (R wave) Thus QR
QS	Yes	Negative	Large	No	–	–	No	–	–	Single large negative deflection is QS
Qr	Yes	Negative	Large	Yes	Positive	Small	No	–	–	First wave is large negative deflection (Q wave), followed by small positive deflection (r wave). Thus Qr

Contd...

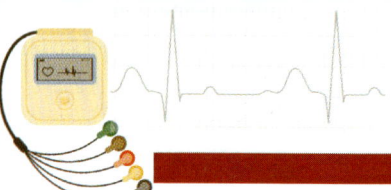

QRS Waveform Types	1st wave			2nd wave			3rd wave			Conclusion
	Present (yes/no)	Deflection (negative/ positive)	Amplitude (large/ small)	Present (yes/no)	Deflection (negative/ positive)	Amplitude (large/ small)	Present (yes/no)	Deflection (negative/ positive)	Amplitude (large/small)	
rsR'	Yes	Positive	small	Yes	Negative	Small	Yes	Positive	Large	First wave is a positive deflection, then a small negative deflection followed by large positive wave. Since negative deflection is below baseline it is designated as S wave. Thus rsR' pattern.
rR'	Yes	Positive	small	Yes	Positive	Large	No	-	-	The negative deflection does not cross the baseline. Thus rR' pattern
qR	Yes	Negative	Large	Yes	Positive	Large	No	–	–	The first negative deflection is small followed by a large R wave. Thus qR
R	Yes	Positive	Large	No	–	–	No	–	–	Notching of R wave upstroke.

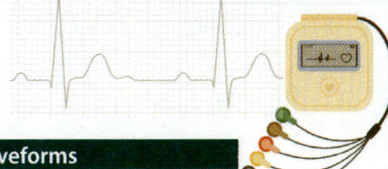

T wave

T wave represents ventricular repolarization. Characteristics of T wave have been described in Table 4.6.

Table 4.6 Characteristics of T wave

Characteristics	• Smooth upright wave, positive in all leads except aVR • It is asymmetrical in shape i.e. its peak is closer to the end of the wave than to the beginning • 1/8 size of R wave • Height <10 mm	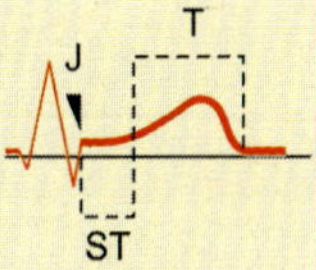
Duration	0.10-0.25 sec	
Abnormality	**Large T waves** Seen in **hyperkalemia** – large, symmetric and pointed wave	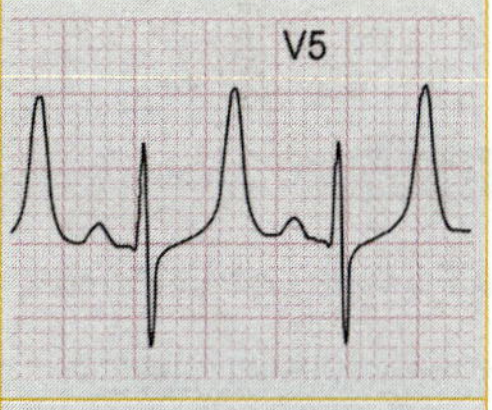 V5
	Negative inverted T waves Seen in post ischemia, acute ischemia, cardiomyopathy (hypertrophic), sometimes with cerebrovascular accidents	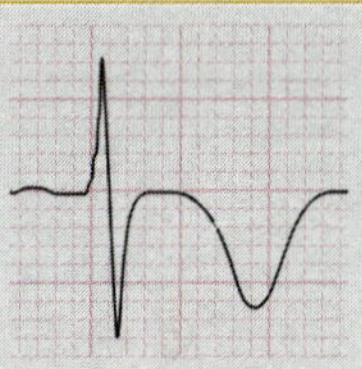
	Flat T waves Hypokalemia or digitalis therapy can cause flattened T wave accompanied with a prominent U wave	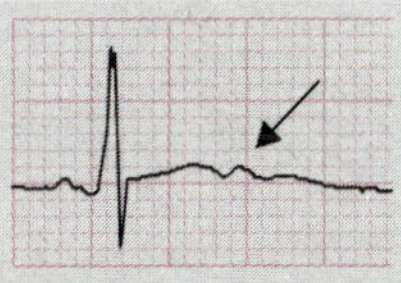 Flat T wave with U wave
	Biphasic T waves **Causes:** Can be seen in myocardial ischemia and hypokalemia.	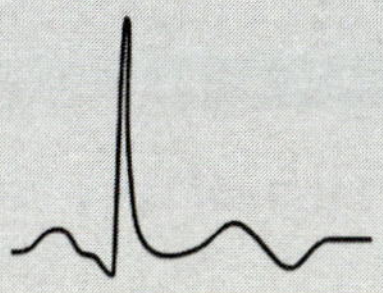
Management	Treatment of underlying disease condition	
Nursing Management	• Check electrolytes specifically K level • Administer treatment as prescribed for hyperkalemia or hypokalemia • Monitor ABG of the patient if hemodynamically unstable or in critical setting • Monitor changes in ECG	

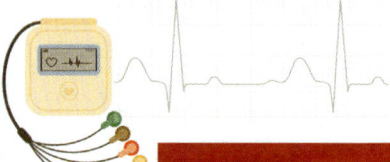

Others

U Wave

- Small, rounded deflection which is sometimes seen after the T wave.
- Prominent U waves are characteristics of hypokalemia (Fig. 4.2).

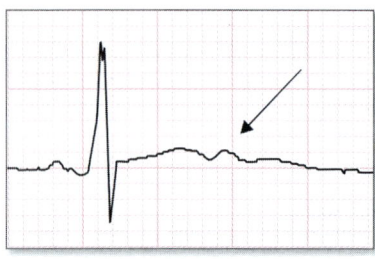

Fig. 4.2 ECG showing U wave

ST Segment Changes

ST segment elevation or depression occurs with myocardial infarction (Figs 4.3A and B).

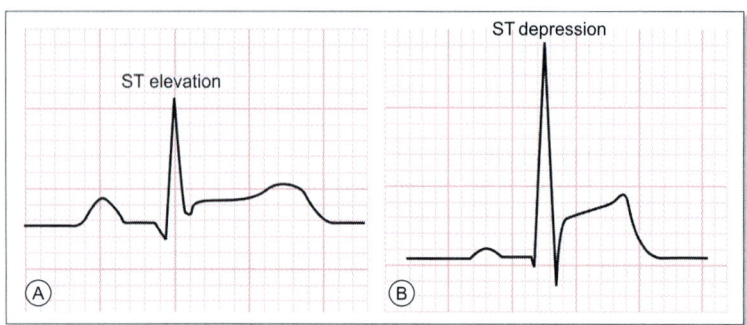

Figs 4.3A and B ECG showing ST segment changes A. ST elevation and B. ST depression

PR Interval

It is associated with AV node blocks, discussed in heart blocks (Chapter 10).

QT Interval

Prolonged QT interval is associated with lethal cardiac arrhythmias, like ventricular fibrillation and torsades de pointes.

Practice Questions

1. Calculate heart rate from the ECG

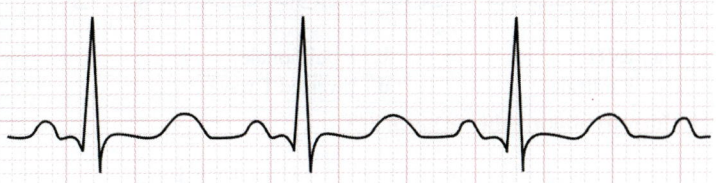

    a. 100 bpm   b. 105 bpm
    c. 107 bpm   d. 110 bpm

2. The given rhythm is –

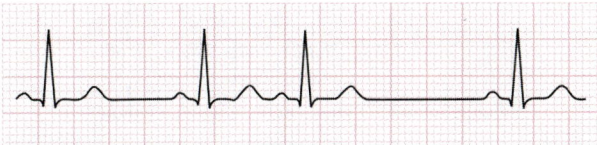

    a. Regular rhythm   b. Irregular rhythm

3. One large box in a ECG grid is equal to

    a. 0.2 sec   b. 0.04 sec
    c. 0.02 sec   d. 0.6 sec

4. One small box in a ECG grid is equal to

    a. 0.2 sec   b. 0.04 sec
    c. 0.02 sec   d. 0.6 sec

5. 6 second strip in an ECG contains:

    a. 15 big box   b. 30 big box
    c. 45 big box   d. 60 big box

6. Identify abnormality in a given ECG

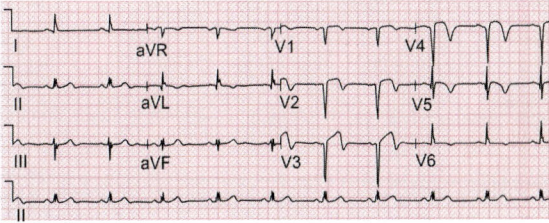

    a. Prolonged PR interval
    b. ST Segment elevation
    c. ST Segment depression
    d. ECG is normal

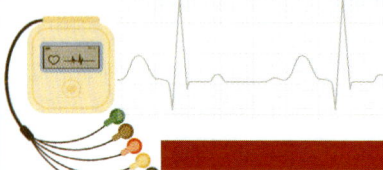
7. Identify abnormality in given ECG

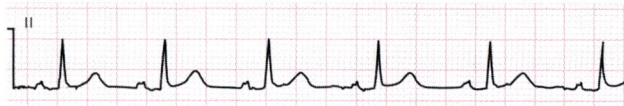

  a. RVH   b. P pulmonale
  c. P mitrale   d. Inverted T wave

8. Identify abnormality in given ECG

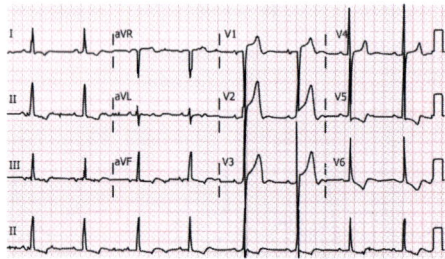

  a. RVH   b. LVH
  c. P mitrale   d. P pulmonale

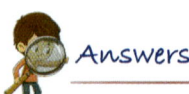

Answers

1. c   2. b   3. a   4. b   5. b
6. b   7. c   8. b

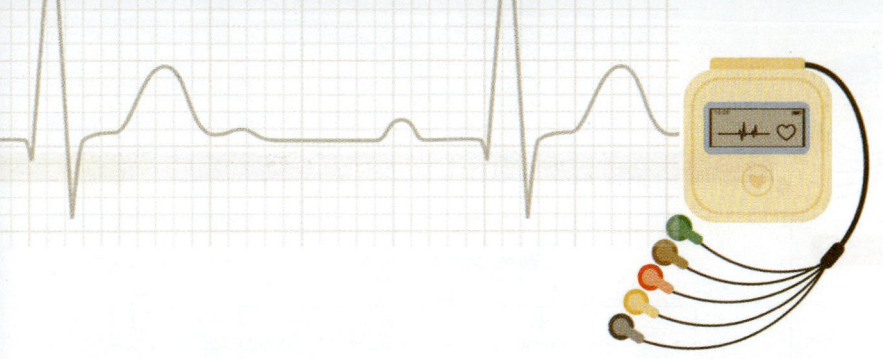

Arrhythmia/ Dysrhythmia

Chapter **5**

INTRODUCTION

The normal heart beats in a regular and coordinated way because electrical impulses are generated and spread by myocytes with unique electrical properties triggering a sequence of organized myocardial contractions. Arrhythmias and conduction disorders are caused by the abnormalities in the generation or conduction of these electrical impulses or both.

Cardiac arrhythmia refers to any change from the normal sequence of electrical impulses. The electrical impulses may happen too fast, too slow, or erratic – causing the heart to beat too fast, too slowly or erratically.

When the heart doesn't beat properly, it can't pump blood effectively. Therefore, arrhythmia affects the cardiac output of the patients and may be fatal in some conditions. Any heart disorder, including congenital abnormalities of structure or function can disturb rhythm. Systemic factors that can cause or contribute to a disturbance in rhythm include: electrolyte abnormalities (particularly potassium, calcium or magnesium), hypoxia, hormonal imbalances (e.g. hypothyroidism, hyperthyroidism), drugs and toxins (e.g. alcohol, caffeine).

CLASSIFICATION OF CARDIAC ARRHYTHMIAS

Arrhythmias can be classified based on various classifications such as:

Based on Site of Origin

- Sinus arrhythmias
- Atrial arrhythmias
- Junctional arrhythmias
- Ventricular arrhythmias

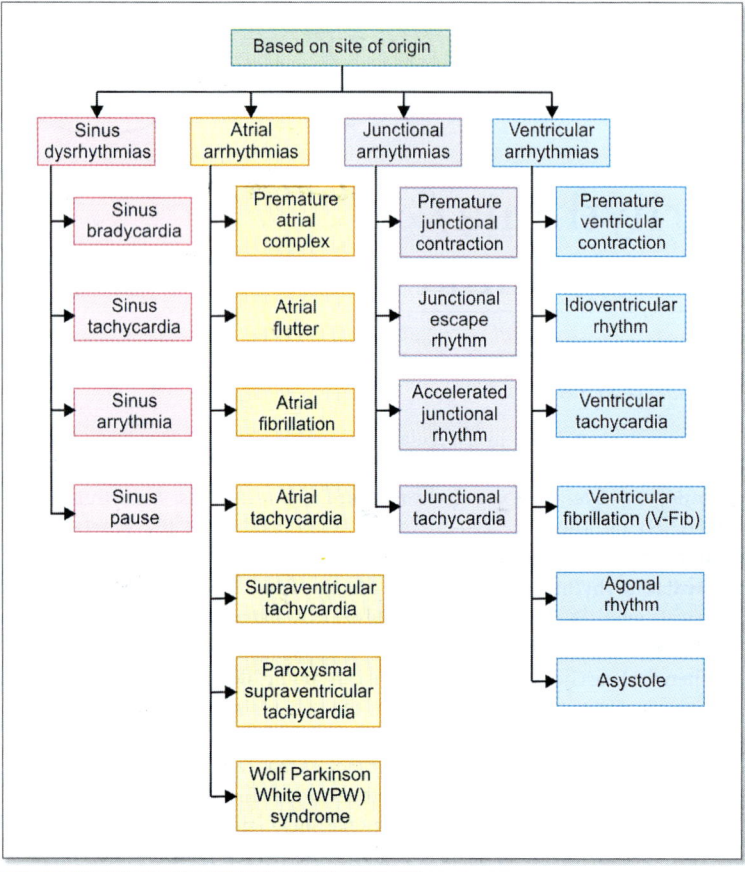

Fig. 5.1 Classification of arrhythmia based on site of origin

Based on Heart Rate

Tachyarrhythmias

Broad-complex tachycardia

- Ventricular fibrillation
- Ventricular tachycardia
- Torsades de Pointes

Narrow-complex tachycardia

- Supraventricular tachyarrhythmias
- Atrial flutter

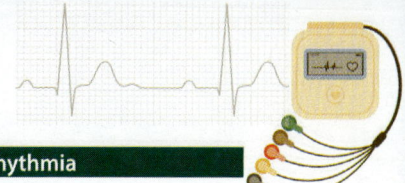

- Atrial fibrillation
- Re-entry supraventricular tachycardia

Bradyarrhythmias

- Heart block
- Bundle branch block

Based on Disorders in Impulse Production and Conduction

Disorders of Impulse Formation

Disturbances of Sinus Mechanism

- Sinus tachycardia
- Sinus bradycardia
- Sinus arrhythmia

Disturbance of Atria

- Atrial premature contraction
- Atrial fibrillation
- Atrial flutter
- Paroxysmal supraventricular tachycardia

Disturbance of Atrioventricular node

- Junctional ectopics
- Junctional rhythm
- Junctional tachycardia

Disturbance of Ventricles

- Ventricular ectopics
- Ventricular tachycardia
- Ventricular fibrillation

Disorders of Impulse Conduction

- Sinoatrial blocks

Atrioventricular (AV) nodal blocks

- First degree block
- Second degree block
  - Wenckebach (Mobitz type I) block
  - Mobitz type II block
  - Complete or third degree block

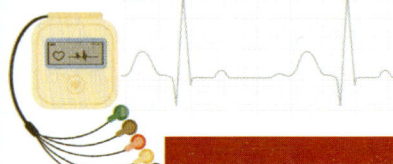

Bundle blocks

- Right bundle branch block
- Left bundle branch block
  - Left anterior hemiblock
  - Left posterior hemiblock

 Practice Questions

1. **Arrhythmias are caused due to:**
   a. Abnormalities in the generation of the electrical impulses
   b. Abnormalities in the conduction of the electrical impulses
   c. Both of the above
   d. None of the above

2. **WPW in WPW syndrome stands for**_____

3. **All of the following are the classification of ventricular arrhythmias except:**
   a. Ventricular tachycardia   b. Agonal rhythm
   c. Idioventricular rhythm   d. Junctional escape rhythm

4. **Which of the following is a type of narrow complex tachycardia:**
   a. Ventricular tachycardia
   b. Ventricular fibrillation
   c. Supraventricular tachycardia
   d. Torsades de points

5. **Another name for Wenckebach block is:**
   a. First degree AV block   b. Mobitz type I block
   c. Mobitz type II block   d. Complete heart block

 Answers

1. **c**
2. **Wolff-Parkinson-White (WPW) syndrome**
3. **d**
4. **c**
5. **b**

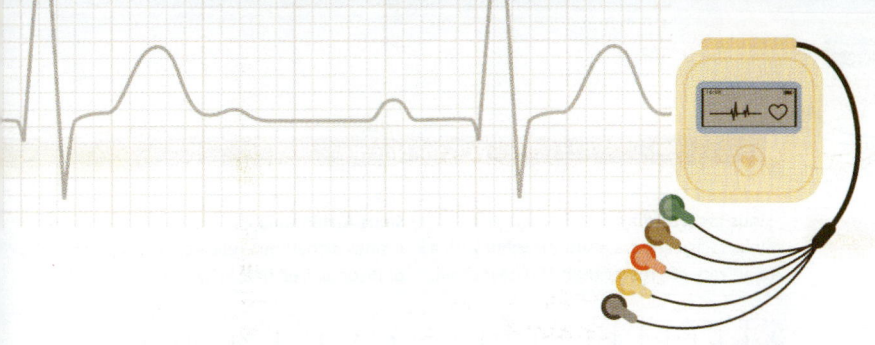

Sinus Rhythms

Chapter 6

INTRODUCTION

Rhythms that originate in the **sinoatrial node** (SA node) are known as **Sinus Rhythms**. In a normally functioning heart, the SA node, also called the sinus node, acts as the **primary pacemaker**. The sinus node assumes this role because its automatic firing rate exceeds that of the heart's other pacemakers. Major identifiable characteristics of sinus rhythm are that the P waves are upright, uniform in appearance and in 1:1 ratio with each QRS.

CLASSIFICATION OF SINUS RHYTHMS (TABLE 6.1)

Sinus rhythms are classified as:
- Normal sinus rhythm (NSR)
- Sinus bradycardia
- Sinus tachycardia
- Sinus arrhythmia
- Sinus pause

Table. 6.1 Types of sinus rhythms

Normal Sinus Rhythm	Sinus Bradycardia
Normal sinus rhythm refers to both a normal heart rate and rhythm.	Sinus bradycardia is sinus rhythm with a heart rate below 60 beats/min.

Contd...

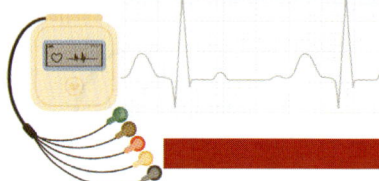

Sinus tachycardia	Sinus Arrhythmia
Sinus tachycardia is a sinus rhythm with a heart rate of greater than 100 beats/min.	A sinus arrhythmia refers to an irregular or disorganized heart rhythm.

Sinus Pause or Arrest

A sinus pause or arrest is defined as the transient absence of sinus P waves that last from 2 seconds to several minutes.

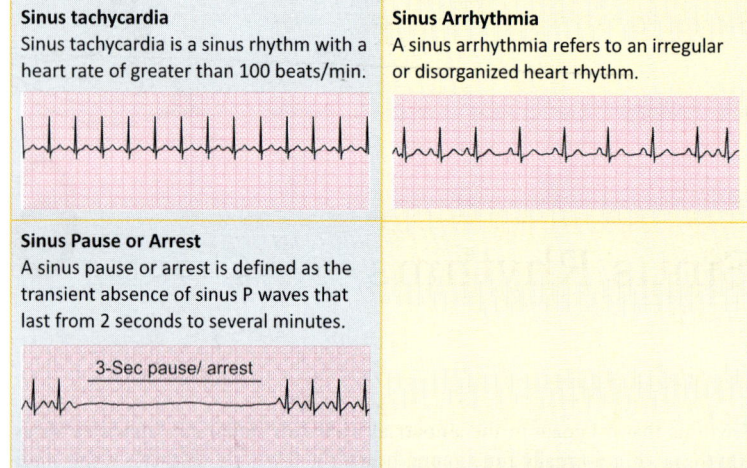

These rhythms are described separately, in subsequent pages.

Normal Sinus Rhythm

NSR is the rhythm that **originates from the sinus node** and describes the characteristic rhythm of the healthy human heart.

NSR is defined as the **rhythm of a healthy heart**.

Key Features

- NSR is the default heart rhythm.
- Pace making impulses arise from the SA node and are transmitted to the ventricles via the AV node and HIS –Purkinje system.
- It is a regular, narrow complex heart rhythm at 60–100 bpm.

Characteristics of NSR have been described in Table 6.2.

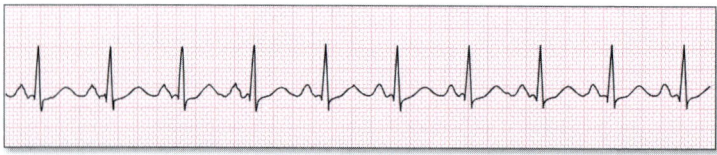

Fig. 6.1 ECG showing normal sinus rhythm

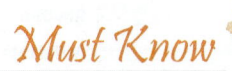

Table 6.2 ECG characteristics of normal sinus rhythm

	Rhythm	Regular
ECG Characteristics (Fig. 6.1)	**Atrial rate**	60-100 beats/min (age appropriate rate in children)
	Ventricular Rate	60-100 beats/min (age appropriate rate in children)
	P wave	Upright in leads I and II, inverted in aVR, duration is <0.12s (<3 small boxes) and amplitude is <2.5 mm.
	P R interval	0.12–0.20s (3–5 small boxes), constant
	QRS complex	Narrow (0.06–0.10s), preceded by a normal P wave
	P: QRS	1:1
	T wave	Upright, sharply or bluntly rounded shape. Duration is 0.10–0.25s, amplitude is <5 mm
	QT interval	0.36–0.44s (9–11 small boxes)
	U wave	Upright and small (0.5 mm), may not always be observed as a result of its small size.

Must Know

- Normal heart rates in children
  - Newborn: 110–150 bpm
  - 2 years: 85–125 bpm
  - 4 years: 75–115 bpm
  - 6 years+: 60–100 bpm
- The lack of normal sinus rhythm is an arrhythmia.

Sinus Bradycardia

Sinus bradycardia is sinus rhythm with a heart rate of below 60 beats/min (Figs 6.2A and B).

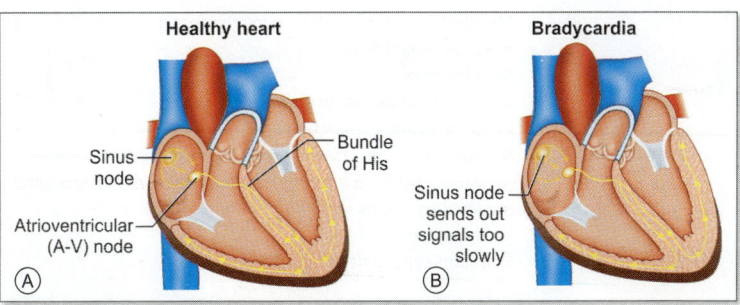

Figs 6.2A and B Changes in heart during bradycardia

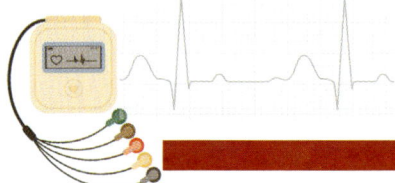

Key Features

- The conduction pathway is the same as that in sinus rhythm but the SA node fires at a rate less than 60 beats/min.
- In sinus bradycardia, decrease in heart rate results from increased vagal stimulation, decreased sympathetic stimulation and/or diminished automaticity in the SA node.

Characteristics of sinus bradycardia have been described in Table 6.3.

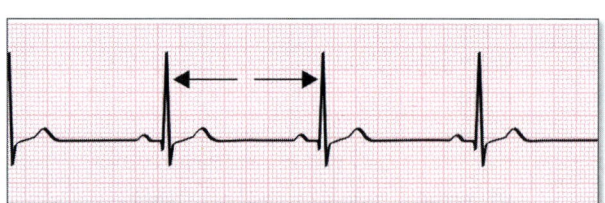

Fig. 6.3 ECG showing sinus bradycardia

Table 6.3 Characteristics of sinus bradycardia

ECG Characteristics (Fig. 6.3)	**Rhythm**	Regular
	Atrial rate	< 60 bpm
	Ventricular Rate	< 60 bpm
	P wave	Before each QRS complex
	P R interval	Normal
	QRS	Normal
	T wave	Normal
	QT interval	Normal
Causes	• **Physiological:** Normal in athletic people • **Iatrogenic:** Beta blockers, calcium channel blockers, anticholinergics, resperine, clonidine, fentanyl, cardiac glycosides. • **Metabolic:** Hyperkalaemia, hypoglycaemia • Increased vagal tone • Hypothermia • Increased intraocular pressure • Acute myocardial infarction • Disease condition – hypothyroidism, increased intracranial pressure, obstructive jaundice, sleep apnea, diphtheria, viral myocarditis, sepsis • Carotid hypersensitivity • Sick sinus syndrome	

Contd...

Signs and Symptoms		• At rest, asymptomatic • Pale, cool and clammy skin • Hypotension • Weakness • Angina • Dizziness or syncope • Confusion and disorientation • Shortness of breath • Light headedness • Exercise intolerance • Chest pain • Decreased cardiac output • Blurred vision

Management	Medical	• Maintenance of airway, breathing and circulation
		• Cardiac monitoring, BP monitoring
		• If the cause of sinus bradycardia is any drug, stop the associated drug.
		• Treatment of cause such as hypothyroidism
		• Treating post infectious bradycardia
		• Administration of medications such as:
		  ▪ Atropine 0.5 mg to I mg, IV/IM (first line drug)
		  ▪ Dopamine: 5 to 20 µg/kg/min
		  ▪ Epinephrine: 2 to 10 µg/min
		  ▪ Isoproterenol: 2 to 10 µg/min
		• Transcutaneous pacing
		• May need permanent pacemaker

	Nursing intervention	• Assess patient – Are they symptomatic?
		• Give oxygen and monitor oxygen saturation
		• Monitor blood pressure and heart rate.
		• Start IV if not already established.
		• Closely monitor the patient especially during discontinuation of medications.
		• Advise the patient for certain lifestyle modifications such as:
		  ▪ Eating a low salt diet
		  ▪ Being active
		  ▪ Getting hypothyroidism treated
		  ▪ Maintaining daily record of pulse rate.

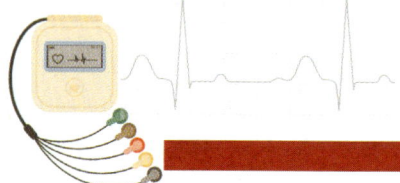

Must Know

- Sinus bradycardia has a clinical association for aerobically trained athletes. Fit individual or aerobically trained athletes have larger stroke volume which means that a greater volume of oxygen is delivered to the body per heartbeat. As exercise and training increases the volume of oxygen that can be delivered to muscles per heart beat, the heart needs to beat less to do the same job. As a result the heart rate is lowered.
- Sick sinus syndrome involves a dysfunction in the ability of SA node to generate or transmit an action potential to the atria which causes bradycardia.

Sinus Tachycardia

Sinus tachycardia is a sinus rhythm with persistence increase in resting heart rate greater than 100 beats/min.

Key Features

- It is normally due to increase in sympathetic activity and/or enhanced automaticity in SA node.
- In sinus tachycardia, discharge rate from the sinus node is increased and conduction pathway remains the same.
- The rate increases gradually and may show beat-to-beat variation but rarely exceeds 140 beats/min in adults (except during heavy exercise).
- Predominantly occurs in women.
- Caused due to enhanced automaticity.

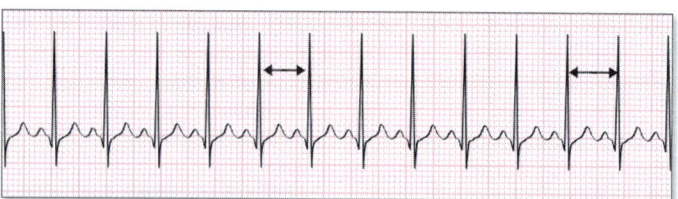

Fig. 6.4 ECG showing sinus tachycardia

Note: On ECG, P wave may be superimposed on preceding T wave and difficult to identify.

Characteristics of sinus tachycardia have been described in Table 6.4.

Table 6.4 Characteristics of sinus tachycardia

ECG Characteristics (Fig. 6.4)	**Rhythm**	Regular
	Atrial rate	>100 beats/min
	Ventricular Rate	>100 beats/min
	P wave	Normal, may become embedded in the preceding T wave
	PR interval	Normal
	QRS	Normal
	P: QRS	1:1
	T wave	Normal
	QT interval	Normal
Causes		• **Physiological causes:** Exertion, exercise, anxiety, pain • **Pathological causes:** Fever, anemia, hypervolemia, hypoxemia, heart failure pulmonary embolism, sepsis, hemorrhage, hypoxia • **Endocrine causes:** Hyperthyroidism, thyrotoxicosis, pheochromocytoma • **Pharmacological causes:** Catecholamine excess, atropine, salbutamol, alcohol, caffeine, nicotine, cocaine
Signs and Symptoms		• Patients intolerance to increased heart rate manifested as palpitations, light headedness, syncope • Dizziness • Dyspnea • Hypotension • Blurred vision • Chest Pain • Anxiety • Nervousness • Crackles if associated with heart failure
Management	**Medical**	• Differentiate whether sinus tachycardia is physiological or pathological • No specific treatment is required for physiological causes, reduce fear and anxiety if present. • In case of pathological sinus tachycardia, treatment is required for underlying cause. • If tachycardia leads to cardiac ischemia, treatment may include beta blockers or calcium channel blockers as they slow the heart rate. • Manage airway, breathing, circulation if needed.

Contd...

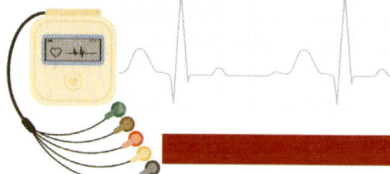

Management	Nursing intervention	• Assess patient:
		  ■ Are they symptomatic?
		  ■ Are they stable?
		• Give oxygen and monitor oxygen saturation.
		• Monitor blood pressure and heart rate.
		• Start IV if not already established.
		• Treat the underlying cause as per the cardiologist's advice, for example:
		  ■ **Fever:** Give acetaminophen or ibuprofen.
		  ■ **Stimulants:** Instruct the patient to stop using caffeine, over the counter (OTC) medications, illicit drugs, etc.
		  ■ **Anxiety:** Give reassurance or anti-anxiety medication
		  ■ Sepsis, anemia, hypotension, myocardial infarction (MI), heart failure, hypoxia need to be treated.

Must Know

- With rapid tachycardia, the P wave may become embedded in the preceding T wave, so the rhythm can be mistaken for atrioventricular nodal tachycardia.
- Recognition of the underlying cause usually facilitates diagnosis of sinus tachycardia. A persistent tachycardia in the absence of an obvious underlying cause should prompt for consideration of atrial flutter or atrial tachycardia.
- Inappropriate sinus tachycardia (IST) is a rare cardiac arrhythmia which can be caused by a malfunction of the autonomic nervous system.

Sinus Arrhythmia

Sinus arrhythmia refers to an irregular or disorganized heart rhythm which can occur without any cause or due to heart damage.

Key Features

Sinus arrhythmia is likely to go undiscovered because it rarely causes symptoms or health issues.

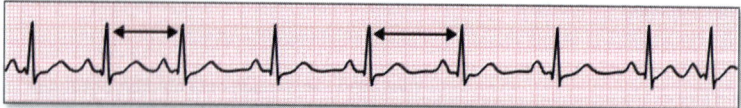

Fig. 6.5 ECG showing sinus arrhythmia

Note: Note the irregularities in rhythm.

Characteristics of sinus arrhythmia have been described in Table 6.5.

Table 6.5 Characteristics of sinus arrhythmia

ECG Characteristics (Fig. 6.5)	**Rhythm**	Irregular (difference varies more than 0.08 sec)
	Atrial rate	Normal
	Ventricular Rate	Normal
	P wave	Normal
	P R interval	Normal
	QRS	Normal
	T wave	Normal
	QT interval	Normal
Causes	• Heart diseases • Moderate to extreme stress • Excessive consumption of stimulants like caffeine, nicotine, and alcohol • Intake of medications like diet pills as well as cough and cold medicines, morphine, etc.	
Sign and Symptom	Patients are usually asymptomatic	
Management	Treatment is usually not required unless the patient is symptomatic. If patient is symptomatic, find and treat the cause.	

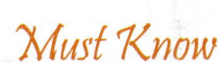

Must Know

Respiratory sinus arrhythmia is a type of sinus arrhythmia, in which the heartbeat changes pace when the person inhales and exhales. In other words, heartbeat cycles change with breath. Breathing in, leads to an increase in heart rate, whereas breathing out causes a drop in heart rate.

During inhalation, the intrathoracic pressure lowers due to contraction and downward movement of the diaphragm which results in expansion of the chest cavity. As a result, atrial pressure also lowers enabling an increased blood flow to the heart. This increase in blood volume towards heart, triggers baroreceptors which act to diminish vagal tone and results in an increased heart rate.

On the opposite during exhalation, diaphragm relaxes, moving upwards which decreases the size of the chest cavity, causing a subsequent increase in the intrathoracic pressure. This increase in pressure inhibits venous return to the heart, resulting in both reduced atrial expansion and minor activation of baroreceptors. As a result, the vagal tone is not suppressed as during inhalation so that it can exert its ability to decrease heart rate (Fig. 6.6).

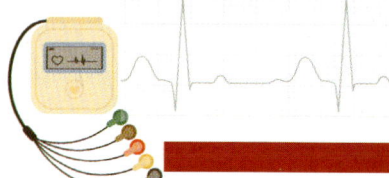
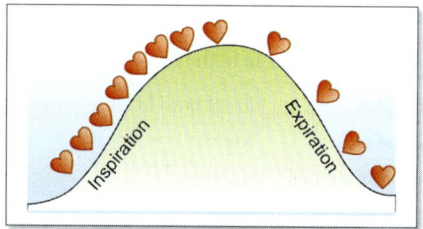

Fig. 6.6 Changes in heart rate during inspiration and expiration

Sinus Arrest or Pause

A sinus pause or arrest is defined as the transient absence of sinus P waves that last from 2 seconds to several minutes which occurs due to sinus node dysfunction.

Key Features

- In sinus arrest or pause, sinus node of the heart transiently ceases to generate the electrical impulses that normally stimulate the myocardial tissues to contract and thus the heart to beat.
- Sinus arrest or pause stimulates parasympathetic system which decreases the SA node automaticity, thereby decreasing heart rate.

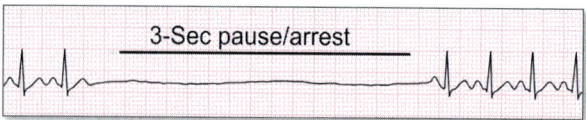

3-Sec pause/arrest

Fig. 6.7 ECG showing sinus pause/arrest

Note: ECG in sinus arrest/pause shows dropped beats in between.

Characteristics of sinus pause/arrest have been described in Table 6.6.

Table 6.6 Characteristics of sinus pause/arrest

ECG Characteristics (Fig. 6.7)	Rhythm	Irregular, when sinus arrest is present
	Atrial rate	Variable, depending on frequency
	Ventricular Rate	Variable, depending on frequency
	P wave	Normal wherever present, may be lost in between
	P R interval	Normal, 0.12–0.20 seconds (3–5 small squares)
	QRS	Normal, 0.06–0.12 seconds (1½ to 3 small squares)
	T wave	Normal
	QT interval	Normal

Contd...

Causes	• **Physiological:**
	  ▪ May occur in individuals with healthy hearts during sleep
	  ▪ Age- elderly
	  ▪ Vagal stimulation
	• **Pathological:**
	  ▪ Myocarditis
	  ▪ Cardiomyopathy
	  ▪ Myocardial infarction (MI)
	  ▪ Digitalis toxicity
	  ▪ Poisoning By grayanotoxin
	  ▪ Hypothyrodisim
	  ▪ Leptospirosis
	  ▪ Pericarditis
	  ▪ Chagas disease
	  ▪ Sarcoidisis
	  ▪ Scleroderma
	  ▪ Diphtheria
	  ▪ Mutation in HCN4 Gene
	  ▪ Cardiac trauma
	  ▪ Erery dreifuss muscular dystrophy
	  ▪ Atrial septal defect
	  ▪ Cannulation of superior vena cava (SVC)
	  ▪ Hyperkalemia

Signs and Symptoms	• Patient may be asymptomatic • Syncope • Dizziness • Loss of consciousness • Bradycardia • Fatigue • Dyspnea on exertion • Palpitations • Light headedness • Chest discomfort
Management	**Medical** • Only treated if patient is symptomatic • Atropine • Pacemaker • In some patients, adenosine administration and carotid sinus massage can also be done • Transesophageal pacing, atrial pacing in pediatric patients **Nursing interventions** • Look for the cause of sinus arrest • Assess patient for BP, heart rate, oxygen saturation. • Teach the patient regarding pacemaker and various do's and don'ts

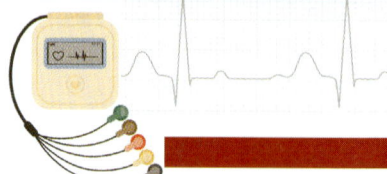

Must Know

- Sinus arrest or sinus pause can also be termed as **Sinoatrial arrest**.
- Medications like beta blockers, digoxin, calcium channel blockers antiarrhythmics, Ivabradine, anticholinestrase inhibitors, lithium, sympathomimetic agents depresses sinus node function which may even lead to sinus arrest or pause.

NURSING PROCESS APPLIED FOR THE PATIENT HAVING SINUS ARRHYTHMIAS

Risk for Decreased Cardiac Output

Nursing Assessment

Tachycardia, hypotension

Nursing Diagnosis

Risk for decreased cardiac output related to altered myocardial contractility which is secondary to arrhythmia as is evidenced by tachycardia and hypotension.

Planning

To maintain normal cardiac output

Nursing Interventions

- Monitor blood pressure and heart rate
- Check capillary refill time
- Assess body temperature of the patient
- Check peripheries for cool and clammy skin
- Obtain 12 lead ECG and interpret the findings
- Start IV, if not already established
- Administer beta blockers or calcium channel blockers as instructed if the cause is sinus tachycardia.

Evaluation

Expected patient outcome may include maintenance of cardiac output and adequate tissue perfusion.

Shortness of Breathing

Nursing Assessment

Dyspnea, restlessness

Nursing Diagnosis

Shortness of breath related to disease condition as evidenced by difficulty in breathing and restlessness.

Planning

To relieve breathing difficulty

Nursing Interventions

- Assess respiratory pattern and pulse rate
- Attach cardiac monitor and check spo2 level of patient
- Administer oxygen through nasal prongs or face mask
- Provide propped up position to the patient
- Obtain 12 lead ECG
- Interpret ECG findings, notify the doctor
- Administer atropine if the cause is sinus bradycardia as per the prescription
- Prepare for transcutaneous pacing as instructed.

Evaluation

Expected patient outcome may include ease in breathing.

Deficient Knowledge about Disease Condition

Nursing Assessment

Patient may look nervous and ask many questions regarding his disease and prognosis.

Nursing Diagnosis

Deficient knowledge related to disease condition as evidenced by frequent questioning by patient.

Planning

- Understanding of disease condition
- Gaining confidence in living with arrrythmias

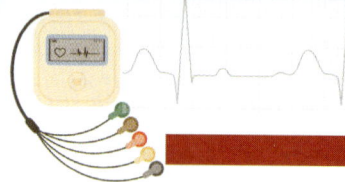

Nursing Interventions

- Explain patient about his/her disease condition in a language easily understood by him/her.
- Reassure the patient and provide support to him/her.
- Instruct to stop using caffeine, over the counter (OTC) medications, illicit drugs, etc.
- Advise for certain lifestyle modifications such as:
  - Eating a low salt diet
  - Being active
  - Getting hypothyroidism treated
  - Maintaining daily record of pulse rate.
- If pacemaker insertion is planned for the patient, explain about the device, its function and associated do's and don'ts (discussed in the annexure).

Evaluation

Expected patient outcomes may include understanding about sinus arrhythmias and gaining confidence for living with arrhythmias.

Practice Questions

1. **Effect of vagal stimulation on heart rate is:**
   - a. Tachycardia
   - b. Bradycardia
   - c. No change

2. **Sinus bradycardia is defined as heart rate:**
   - a. Below 30 b/min
   - b. Below 40 b/min
   - c. Below 50 b/min
   - d. Below 60 b/min

3. **Sinus arrhythmia is characterized by:**
   - a. Abnormal P wave morphology
   - b. Irregular rhythm
   - c. Abnormal rate
   - d. Abnormal QRS morphology

4. **The arrhythmia which is normally present in athletes is:**
   - a. Sinus tachycardia
   - b. Sinus bradycardia
   - c. Sinus pause
   - d. None of the above

5. **With inspiration HR_____and with expiration HR_____.**
   - a. Increases, decreases
   - b. Increases, increases
   - c. Decreases, increases
   - d. Decreases, decreases

6. **All of the following medications may cause sinus pause except:**
   - a. Ivabradine
   - b. Atropine
   - c. Beta blockers
   - d. Digoxin

7. **P wave may embed in preceding T wave in which of the following arrhythmia:**
   - a. Sinus bradycardia
   - b. Sinus tachycardia
   - c. Sinus arrhythmia
   - d. Sinus Pause

8. **Treatment of asymptomatic bradycardia is:**
   - a. Atropine
   - b. Isoprenaline
   - c. Cardiac pacing
   - d. No treatment is required

9. **Identify the rhythm**

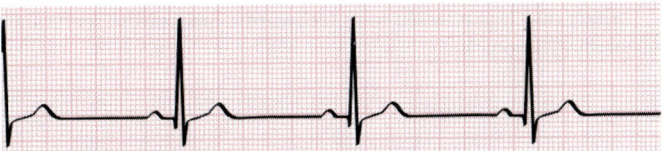

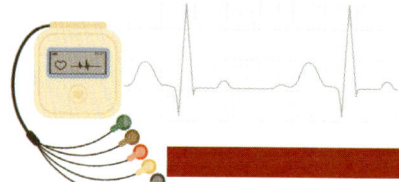

10. Identify the rhythm

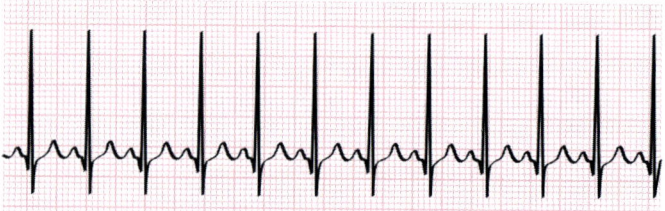

11. Identify the rhythm

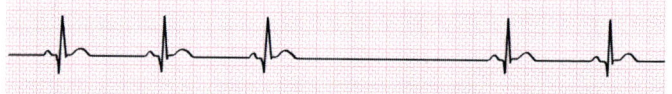

12. Identify the rhythm

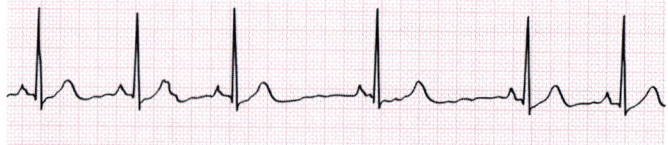

13. Identify the rhythm

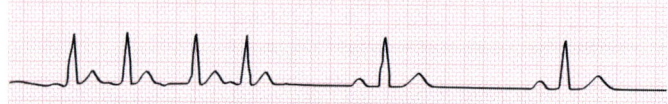

Ans. Tachycardia-bradycardia syndrome. It is a type of sick sinus syndrome which is characterized by a brief irregular tachycardia followed by slow sinus node discharge.

Explanation: Sick sinus syndrome (SSS) refers to the dysfunction of the sinoatrial node and is responsible for several types of arrhythmia. It comprises bradyarrhythmias (e.g., sinus bradycardia, sinoatrial pauses, blocks, and arrest) and may alternate with supraventricular tachyarrhythmias, in which case it is referred to as tachycardia-bradycardia syndrome (tachy brady syndrome).

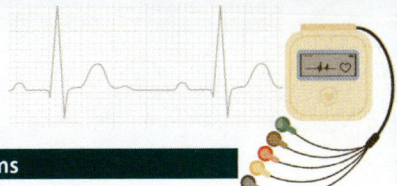

Types of Sick Sinus Syndrome

1.	Sinoatrial block	Electrical signals move too slowly through the sinus node, causing an abnormally slow heart rate.
2.	Sinus arrest	The sinus node activity pauses, causing skipped beats.
3.	Bradycardia-tachycardia syndrome	The heart rate alternates between abnormally fast and slow rhythms, usually with a long pause (asystole) between heartbeats.

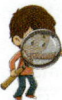 Answers

1.	b	2.	d	3.	b	4.	b
5.	a	6.	b	7.	b	8.	d

9. Sinus bradycardia
10. Sinus tachycardia
11. Sinus pause
12. Sinus arrhythmia
13. Tachycardia-bradycardia syndrome.

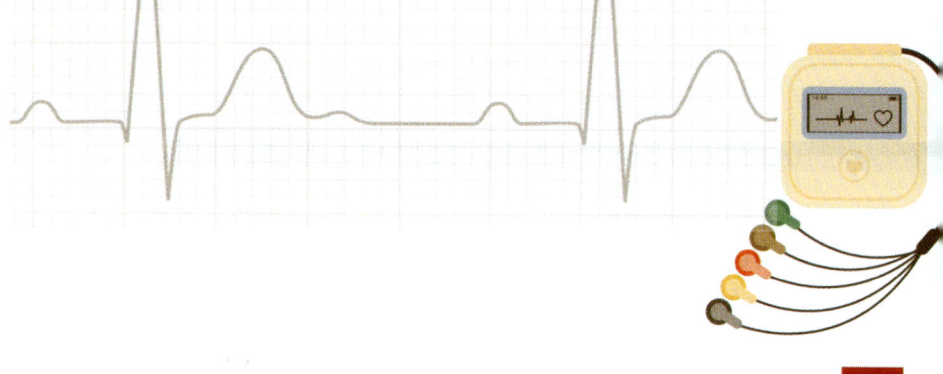

Atrial Rhythms

Chapter 7

INTRODUCTION

- Atrial rhythms **originate in the atria** rather than in the sinoatrial (SA) node. The P wave will be positive, but its shape can be different than a normal sinus rhythm because the electrical impulse follows a different path to the atrioventricular (AV) node.
- When the SA node fails to generate an impulse; atrial tissues or internodal pathways may initiate an impulse.
- Atrial dysrhythmias reflect abnormal electrical impulse formation (also called automatic) or abnormal conduction (also called reentrant) in the atria.

CLASSIFICATION OF ATRIAL ARRHYTHMIAS (TABLE 7.1)

Broadly atrial arrhythmias can be divided into following main sub classifications:
- Premature atrial complex
- Atrial flutter
- Atrial fibrillation
- Atrial tachycardia
- Supraventricular tachycardia
- Multifocal atrial tachycardia
- Paroxysmal supraventricular tachycardia (PSVT)
- Wolf parkinson white (WPW) syndrome

Table 7.1 Classification of atrial arrhythmias

Premature atrial complex	Atrial flutter
This occurs when an ectopic site within the atria fires an impulse before the next impulse from the SA node.	Atrial flutter is characterized by 'sawtooth' appearance of P waves and occurs when an irritable site in the atria generates impulses at an extremely rapid rate and over-rides the SA node as pacemaker.

Contd...

Atrial fibrillation
This occurs when irritable sites in the atria fire at rate faster than 400 times a minute. The muscle quivers, resulting in ineffectual atrial contraction.

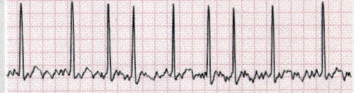

Atrial tachycardia
This occurs when an irritable area of the atria fires impulses faster than the SA Node and becomes the pacemaker for the heart.

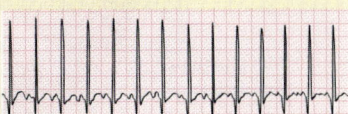

Supraventricular tachycardia
This covers three types of tachycardia that originate in the atria, AV junction or SA node.

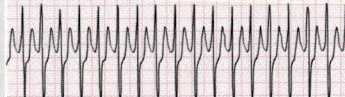

Multifocal atrial tachycardia
Multiple (non-SA) sites fire impulses in multifocal atrial tachycardia. The P waves will vary in shape and at least three different shapes can be observed. The PR Interval varies. Ventricular rhythm is irregular.

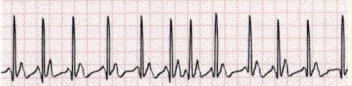

Paroxysmal supraventricular tachycardia (PSVT)
Supraventricular tachycardia that starts or ends very suddenly is called paroxysmal supraventricular tachycardia (PSVT).

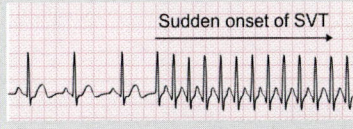

Sudden onset of SVT

Wolf Parkinson White (WPW) syndrome
In WPW an accessory conduction pathway is present between the atria and the ventricles. Electrical impulses are rapidly conducted to the ventricles. These rapid impulses create a slurring of the initial portion of the QRS called the delta wave.

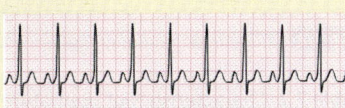

These rhythms are described separately, in subsequent pages.

Premature Atrial Contractions (Fig. 7.1)

Premature atrial contractions are common cardiac dysrhythmias characterized by premature heartbeats originating in the atria.

PACs are extra beats that originate outside the sinus node somewhere in the atria.

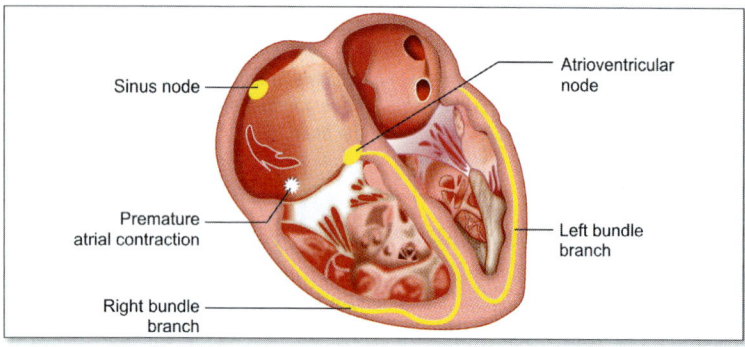

Fig. 7.1 Diagrammatic representation of premature atrial contraction

Key Features

- PACs occur when another region of the atria (other than SA node) depolarizes before the SA node and thus triggers a premature heartbeat.
- If the ectopic site is near the SA node, the P wave will likely have a shape similar to a sinus rhythm. But this P wave will occur earlier than expected.
- Simply stated, PAC is a normal beat, but just occurs early.
- P wave may have different morphology on ectopic beat, but it will be present.

Characteristics of PACs have been described in Table 7.2.

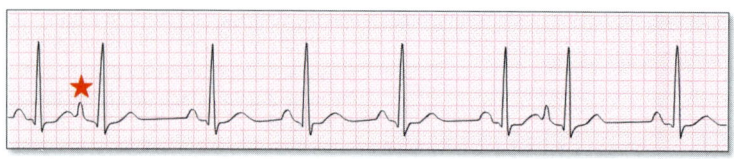

Fig. 7.2 ECG showing premature atrial contractions

Table 7.2 Characteristics of premature atrial contraction

ECG Characteristics (Fig. 7.2)	**Rhythm**	Irregular when PACs occur. The baseline rhythm is regular.
	Atrial rate	Usually normal but depends on underlying rhythm
	Ventricular rate	Usually normal but depends on underlying rhythm
	P wave	Premature P wave with an abnormal configuration and may be lost in the previous T wave
	PR interval	Normal, shortened, or slightly prolonged, depending on the origin of the ectopic focus
	QRS	Normal
	T wave	Abnormal with some embedded P waves
	QT interval	Normal

Contd...

Causes	• Can be triggered by alcohol, nicotine, caffeine, cigarette, anxiety or fatigue. • Coronary or valvular heart disease • Acute respiratory failure • Hypoxia • Pulmonary disease • Myocardial infarction • Beta agonists • Sympathomimetics • Digoxin toxicity • Certain electrolyte imbalances such as hypokalaemia, and hypomagnaesemia.	
Signs and Symptoms	Most of the time PACs cause no symptoms and can go unrecognized for years. The patient may perceive PACs as normal palpitations or skipped beats. Symptoms depend on frequency of PACs. When the PACs occur, patient may have: • Irregular heart beat • Hypotension • Pulse deficit • Syncope • Fluttering sensation	
Management	**Medical**	• Asymptomatic patients don't need treatment. In symptomatic patients, however, treatment may focus on eliminating the cause. • Remove stimulants • Correct electrolyte imbalance if this is the cause. • If the patient has ischemic or valvular heart disease, monitor him for signs and symptoms of heart failure, electrolyte imbalances, and the development of more severe atrial arrhythmias.
	Nursing	Teach patient to: • Eliminate the cause, such as caffeine, alcohol, and nicotine. • Learn stress reduction techniques to lessen his/her anxiety.

Must Know

• A PAC is not a rhythm, it is an ectopic beat that originates from the atria.
• PACs are also known as atrial premature complexes (APC) or atrial premature beats (APB).
• If no QRS complex follows the premature P wave, a non-conducted PAC occurs.
• A non-conducted PAC (Fig. 7.3), however, is an atrial impulse that arrives early to the AV node, when the node isn't yet repolarized. As a result, the premature P wave fails to be conducted to the ventricle.
• PACs may occur in bigeminy (every other beat is a PAC), trigeminy (every third beat is a PAC), or couplets (two PACs in a row).

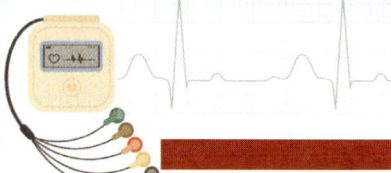

Nonconducted PAC

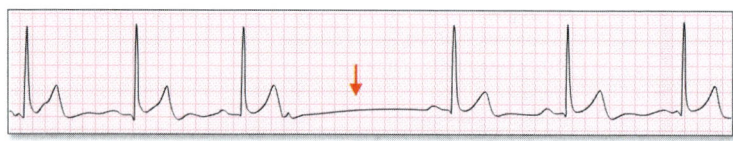

Fig. 7.3 ECG showing Nonconducted PAC

Atrial Tachycardia

In atrial tachycardia, **electrical impulse comes from an ectopic pacemaker**, i.e. from the atria rather than from the SA node Fig. 7.4.

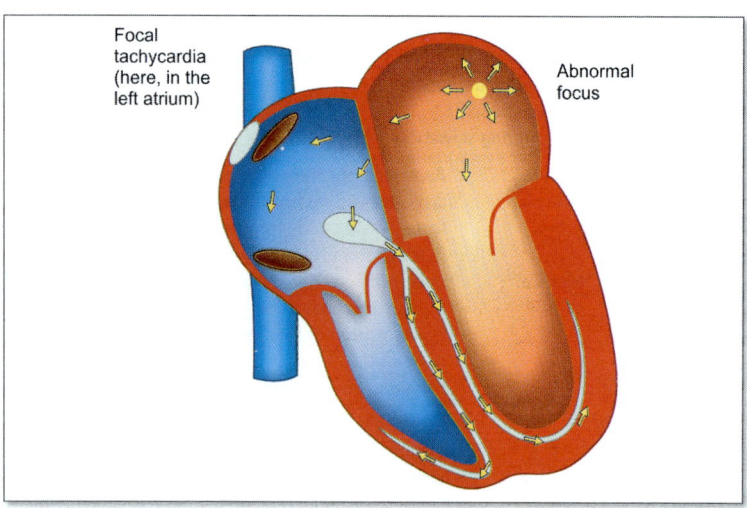

Focal tachycardia (here, in the left atrium)

Abnormal focus

Fig. 7.4 Diagrammatic representation of atrial tachycardia in left atrium

Key Features

- The rapid rate resulting from atrial tachycardia shortens diastole, resulting in a loss of atrial kick, reduced cardiac output, reduced coronary perfusion and ischemic myocardial changes.
- It is characterized by three or more successive ectopic atrial beats at a rate of 150 to 250 beats/minute.
- Atrial tachycardia can have a right or left origin.

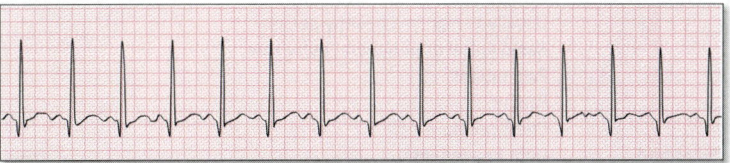

Fig. 7.5 ECG showing atrial tachycardia

Characteristic of atrial tachycardia have been described in Table 7.3.

Table 7.3 Characteristics of atrial tachycardia

	Rhythm	Atrial rhythm: regular ventricular rhythm is regular when the block is constant and irregular, when it isn't.
ECG Characteristics (Fig. 7.5)	**Atrial rate**	150 to 250 beats/minute
	Ventricular rate	Varies according to the AV conduction ratio
	P wave	May not be discernible and may be hidden in the previous ST segment or T wave.
	PR interval	Can't measure
	QRS	Normal
	P:QRS	1:1 unless a block is present
	T wave	Distorted by P wave
	QT interval	Normal or Less than normal

Causes		• Can be in normal adults with excessive use of caffeine or other stimulants, marijuana use, due to exercise and physical or psychological stress.
		• May also be due to an associated cardiac condition such as:
		  ▪ Myocardial dial infarction
		  ▪ Cardiomyopathy
		  ▪ Congenital anomalies
		  ▪ Wolff-Parkinson-White Syndrome
		  ▪ Valvular heart disease
		  ▪ Corpulmonale
		  ▪ Sick sinus syndrome
		  ▪ Systemic hypertension and digoxin toxicity
		• May also be due to
		  ▪ Chronic obstructive pulmonary disease (COPD)
		  ▪ Altered fluid status
		  ▪ Excessive catecholamine release
		  ▪ Hyperthyroidism
		  ▪ Hypoxia
		  ▪ Electrolyte imbalances (hypokalaemia and hypomagnaesemia)

Contd...

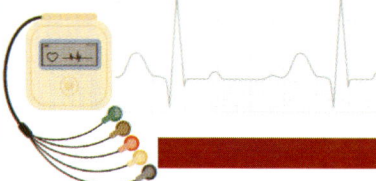
Signs and Symptoms		• Usually benign in a healthy person • Rapid apical or peripheral pulse rate • Palpitations • Fatigue • Chest pressure • Light headedness • Blurred vision • Syncope • Dyspnea • Hypotension • May lead to angina, heart failure, ischemic myocardial changes, and even MI and symptoms may progress accordingly.
Management	**Medical**	• Vagal maneuvers such as Valsalva's maneuver or carotid sinus massage • Drugs such as digoxin, beta-adrenergic blockers, and calcium channel blockers. • Atrial overdrive pacing (atrial pacing at an increased lower rate, exceeding the patient's mean intrinsic rate.)
	Nursing intervention	If vagal maneuvers are used, make sure that resuscitative equipment is readily available as these can result in bradycardia, ventricular arrhythmias, and asystole.

Table 7.4 Types of Atrial Tachycardia

Multifocal Atrial Tachycardia (MAT)	Paroxysmal Atrial Tachycardia (PAT)
In MAT, atrial tachycardia occurs with numerous atrial foci firing intermittently. ↓ MAT produces varying P waves on the strip and occurs most commonly in patients with chronic pulmonary disease. (Wandering atrial pacemaker is an irregular rhythm. It is similar to multifocal atrial tachycardia but the heart rate is under 100 bpm. P waves are present but will vary in shape.) 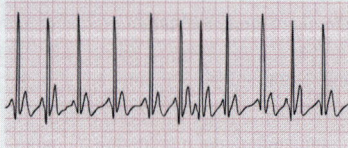	PAT is a type of paroxysmal supraventricular tachycardia, in which there are brief periods of tachycardia that alternate with periods of normal sinus rhythm. ↓ PAT starts and stops suddenly as a result of rapid firing of an ectopic focus. ↓ It commonly follows frequent PACs, one of which initiates the tachycardia. 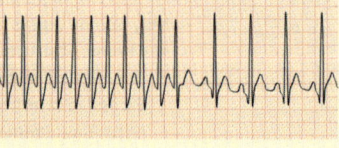

Must Know

There are three types of atrial tachycardia: atrial tachycardia with block, multifocal atrial tachycardia, and paroxysmal atrial tachycardia (PAT).
- Atrial tachycardia with an atrioventricular block is typically seen with digoxin toxicity.
- Paroxysmal atrial tachycardia (PAT) is also known as focal atrial tachycardia.
- Atrial overdrive pacing may also be used to stop the arrhythmia. This treatment helps suppress the depolarization of the ectopic pacemaker and permits the SA node to resume its normal role.
- Carotid sinus massage must not be performed on older patients.

Atrial Flutter (Fig. 7.6)

Atrial flutter is characterized by large **re-entry circuit within the right atrium**, usually encircling the tricuspid annulus.

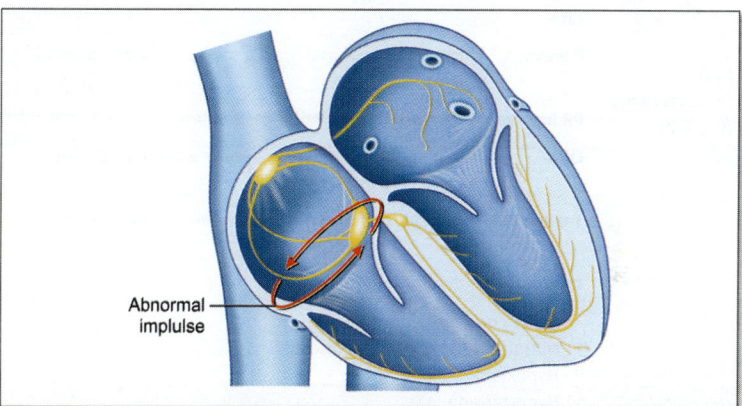

Abnormal impulse

Fig. 7.6 Re-entry circuit In Atrial Flutter

Key Features

- **"Impulses take a circular course around the atria, setting up the flutter waves"**
- AV node conducts impulses to the ventricles at a 2:1, 3:1, 4:1, or greater ratio (rarely 1:1).
- Flutter waves have a saw-tooth appearance.
- The presence of A-flutter may be the first indication of cardiac disease.

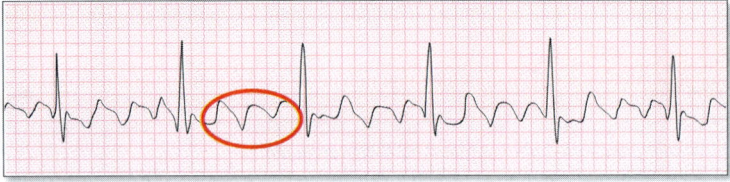

Fig. 7.7 ECG showing atrial flutter

Note: ECG shows multiple P waves followed by QRS complex that may be in the ratio of 2:1, 3:1 or 4:1.

Characteristic of atrial flutter have been described in Table 7.5.

Table 7.5 Characteristics of atrial flutter

ECG Characteristics (Fig. 7.7)	**Rhythm**	Usually regular but may be variable
	Atrial rate	250–350 bpm
	Ventricular rate	Variable (slow or fast)
	P wave	Obscured by flutter waves, sawtooth appearance of P waves
	PR interval	Variable (usually not measurable)
	QRS	Usually normal but may appear widened if flutter waves are buried in QRS
	T wave	Difficult to differentiate between T wave and flutter waves
	QT interval	Cannot measure
Causes	<ul><li>Acute coronary syndrome</li><li>Mitral and tricuspid valve disorders</li><li>Hypoxia</li><li>Hypertension</li><li>Chronic lung disease</li><li>Cardiomyopathy</li><li>Pulmonary embolus and corpulmonale</li><li>Hyperthyroidism</li><li>Obesity</li><li>Alcohol consumption</li><li>Diabetes</li><li>Pheochromocytoma</li><li>Electrolyte imbalance</li><li>Drug induced (antiarrhythmic drugs and digitalis toxicity)</li></ul>	

Contd...

Signs and Symptoms		• Palpitations and dyspnoea induced by even slight physical exercise. • On physical examination, the pulse is rapid and more frequently regular than irregular. • Patient may have exercise intolerance. • Hypotension and fainting may also occur.
Management	Medical	• Adenosine, amiodarone, beta adrenergic blocking agents, calcium channel antagonists and digitalis slow the ventricular rate by increasing atrio ventricular block. However, the most effective method is electrical cardioversion, which produces sinus rhythm in almost all patients with atrial flutter (restoration of sinus rhythm). • Catheter ablation of the re-entrant circuit with radiofrequency current can also be done (Radiofrequency ablation, RFA). • Antiarrhythmic drugs can also be considered in patients with symptomatic recurrent atrial flutter. • Patients with persistent flutter should receive chronic anticoagulation to prevent the formation of emboli.
	Nursing	• Drugs may lead to hypotension, dizziness, and syncope therefore, safety measures are important to take. • Monitor vital signs of the patient. • Prepare for cardioversion. • Check aPTT, PT, INR of the patient if on anticoagulant therapy. • Educate the patients regarding self–management if on anticoagulant therapy.

Types of Atrial Flutter

Atrial flutter can further be divided into following subtypes:

- **Type I (also called classical or typical)** has a rate of 250-350 bpm.
- **Type II (also called non-typical)** are faster, ranging from 350-450 bpm.

Or

- **Paroxysmal atrial flutter:** Atrial flutter which comes and goes. An episode of atrial flutter usually lasts for hours or days.
- **Persistent atrial flutter:** This type of atrial flutter is more or less permanent.

Must Know

The AV node has a refractory period that prevents it from conducting impulses at more than about 230/min. This results in a degree of atrioventricular block, commonly 2:1 or 3:1 and in a ventricular rate of a half or one third of the atrial rate, typically 150 beats/min.

- Flutter may be paroxysmal, in this case there is usually a precipitating factor such as pericarditis or acute respiratory failure, or it may be persistent.
- If AV node blocks the impulses at a regular rate, the ventricular rate will be regular. If the AV node blocks the impulses at an irregular rate, the ventricular rate will be irregular. Atrial flutter is characterized by no identifiable p-waves, replaced by a "sawtooth" flutter.
- Antiarrhythmic drugs can paradoxically induce dysrhythmias as well, including atrial fibrillation and atrial flutter by influencing the electrical properties of the atrial myocardium.

Difference between Atrial Flutter and Atrial Fibrillation

It is important to understand the difference between atrial flutter and fibrillation.

Atrial flutter is more temporary as compared to atrial fibrillation. If atrial flutter lasts for more than a week it may convert into atrial fibrillation. Rhythm is regular in atrial flutter and irregular in atrial fibrillation. And also complication such as systemic embolization are less common with atrial flutter as compared to atrial fibrillation.

Atrial Fibrillation (Figs 7.8A and B)

Atrial fibrillation, sometimes called AF or A fib, is defined as chaotic, asynchronous, electrical activity in atrial tissue.

In atrial fibrillation, a multiple rapid impulse from many foci depolarize in the atria in a totally disorganized manner at a rate of 350 to 600 beats/minute.

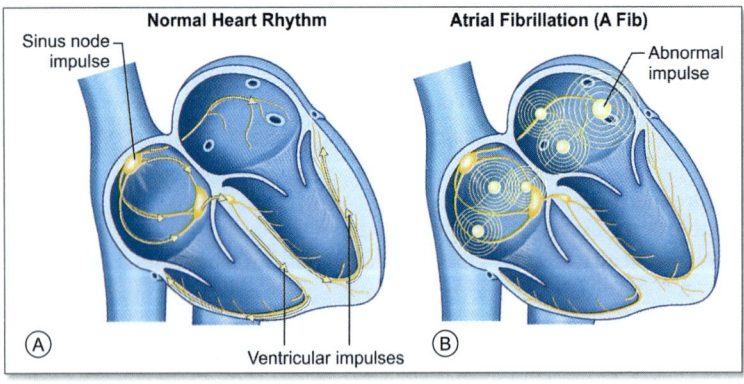

Figs 7.8A and B (A) Normal heart rhythm; (B) Atrial fibrillation

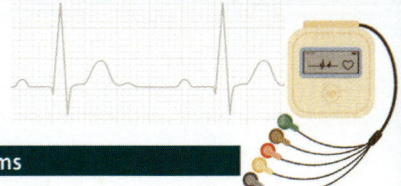

Key Features

- In AF, an impulse is generated by multiple sites within the atria.
- Absent P wave which is replaced by fibrillating F wave.
- Rhythm is irregularly, irregular.
- Presence of multiple, interacting re-entry circuit looping around the atria.
- Total disorganization of atrial electrical activity due to multiple ectopic foci resulting in loss of effective atrial contraction.
- Atria quiver which lead to formation of thrombi.

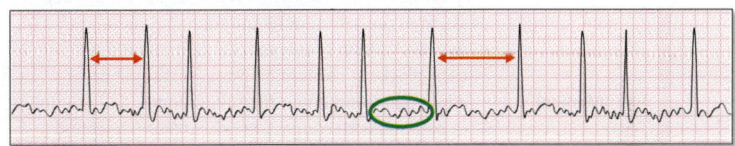

Fig. 7.9 ECG showing atrial fibrillation

Characteristics of atrial fibrillation haven been described in Table 7.6.

Table 7.6 Characteristics of atrial fibrillation

ECG Characteristics (Fig. 7.9)	**Rhythm**	Irregular
	Atrial rate	350 bpm or greater
	Ventricular rate	Slow or fast, variable
	P wave	Absent
	PR interval	Cannot differentiate
	QRS	Normal
	T wave	Indiscernible (indistinguishable)
	QT interval	Cannot measure
Causes	<ul><li>Thyrotoxicosis</li><li>Alcohol intoxication</li><li>Caffeine use</li><li>Electrolyte disturbance (hypokalaemia, hypocalcaemia and hypomagnaesemia)</li><li>Stress</li><li>Advancing age</li><li>Cardiac surgery</li><li>Cardiac conditions such as rheumatic heart disease (RHD), valvular insufficiencies, myocarditis, atrial ischemia</li><li>May occur without any underlying heart disease and known as idiopathic or Lone AFib.</li></ul>	

Contd...

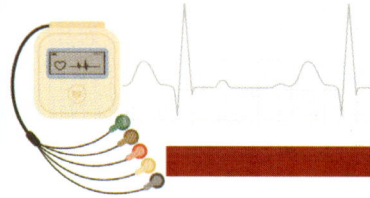

Signs and Symptoms		• 90% AF do not cause sign and symptoms
		• Patients may have:
		  ▪ Irregular pulse ▪ Pulse deficit
		  ▪ Fatigue, angina, dyspnea ▪ Palpitation, dizziness, syncope

Manage-ment	Medical	• Haemodynamically unstable atrial fibrillation with a rapid ventricular rate of (> 120 beats/min): Immediate electrical cardioversion regardless of the duration of the arrhythmia.
		• Maintenance of airway, breathing and circulation.
		• Stable, rapid atrial fibrillation (ventricular rate of >120 beats/min) regardless of its duration:
		  ▪ In patients with preserved left ventricular function: beta-blockers, calcium blockers (verapamil or diltiazem) and digitalis (first line agent).
		  ▪ In patients with congestive heart failure, (ejection fraction of < 40%): digitalis, diltiazem, and amiodarone.
		• Anti-coagulants for the prevention of systemic embolisation.
		• In case of failure of pharmacological measures: Non-pharmacologic strategies such as pacemakers, atrial defibrillators, catheter ablation for either rate control or prevention of atrial fibrillation, and surgery should be considered.

	Nursing	• Prescribed medications may affect the cardiovascular system, leading to haemodynamic changes, such as hypotension, dizziness, and syncope, so safety measures are important. • If the patient is taking anticoagulants, then lab values [activated partial thromboplastin time (aPTT) for heparin, prothrombin time (PT), international normalized ration (INR) for warfarin] as well as signs of bleeding and vital signs especially BP should be monitored. • Prepare for cardioversion. Prior to cardioversion sedation medication and/or analgesics should be given for client comfort. The nurse would administer and monitor the effects of analgesia. • Nurses should check with their institution for policies and procedures related to nursing responsibilities when conscious sedation is used as commonly used during cardioversion. • After the procedure, monitor the chest wall for burns, and medicate for pain as ordered. A patient may have a sore chest after synchronized cardioversion, so providing comfort measures, such as repositioning, mild analgesic, and warm compresses to the chest, may assist in easing the discomfort. • Long term monitoring of patients is required.

Must Know

- Afib is a leading cause of strokes as in atrial fibrillation, the "atrial kick" is lost and cardiac output decreases. As blood pools in the atria, clots may form and cause serious damage due to embolism or embolic episodes (such as stroke). For this reason, patients are placed on anticoagulant therapy.
- Afib can fly under the radar as some patients don't have symptoms and some may only have symptoms once in a while. Thus, patients may go for a year or two undiagnosed and sometimes not be diagnosed until after they have a stroke or two.
- Afib is one of the most common arrhythmia of elderly.
- If a patient has Afib with acute heart failure exacerbations, calcium channel blockers and beta blockers should be avoided as they are negative ionotropes.

Supraventricular Tachycardia (Figs 7.10A and B)

- Supraventricular tachycardia (SVT) is a rapid heart rate that is caused by electrical impulses which originate above the heart's ventricles.
- Encompasses all fast (tachy) dysrhythmias in which heart rate is greater than 150 beats per minute (bpm).
- SVT is triggered by reentry mechanism.

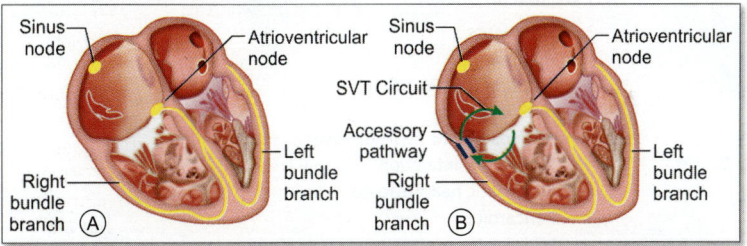

Figs 7.10A and B (A) Normal electrical conduction; (B) Supraventricular tachycardia

Key Features

- There are four main types: atrial fibrillation, paroxysmal supraventricular tachycardia (PSVT), atrial flutter, and Wolff–Parkinson–White syndrome.
- SVT, is often used synonymously with AV nodal re-entry tachycardia (AVNRT).
- In SVT, narrow QRS complex occur, although, occasionally, there may be wide QRS complex that may mimic ventricular tachycardia (VT).

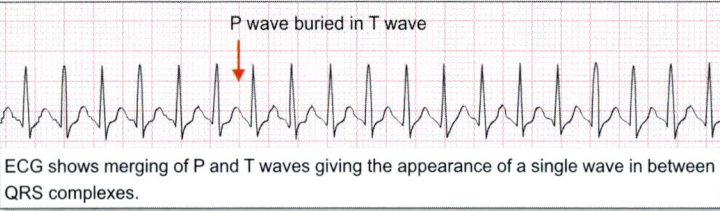

P wave buried in T wave

ECG shows merging of P and T waves giving the appearance of a single wave in between QRS complexes.

Fig. 7.11 ECG showing supraventricular tachycardia

Characteristics of supraventricular tachycardia have been described in Table 7.7.

Table 7.7 Characteristics of supraventricular tachycardia

ECG Characteristics (Fig. 7.11)	**Rhythm**	Regular
	Atrial rate	150-250 bpm
	Ventricular rate	150-250 bpm
	P wave	Becomes hidden in the QRS
	PR interval	Usually not discernable
	QRS	Normal
	T wave	P wave and T wave are merged together
	QT interval	Short
Causes	• Stimulants • Hypoxia • Stress or over-exertion • Hypokalaemia • Atherosclerotic heart disease • Myocardial infarction • Rheumatic heart disease • Pericarditis • Mitral valve prolapse • Chronic lung disease • Hyperthyroidism • Thyrotoxicosis	
Signs and Symptoms	• Palpitations • Chest discomfort (pressure, tightness, pain) • Lightheadedness or dizziness • Syncope • Shortness of breath • A pounding pulse • Sweating • Nausea • Tightness or fullness in the throat • Tiredness (fatigue) • Excessive urine production	

Contd...

| Management | Medical | • Stable patient's (asymptomatic)
  ■ Vagal maneuvers
• Drug management
  ■ Adenosine
  ■ Calcium channel blockers
• Cardioversion if unstable (most effective)
• Carotid sinus massage |
| | Nursing | • Assess Patient
• Administer O_2
• Vagal maneuvers (cough and valsalva)
• Start intravenous if not already established
• Prepare for cardioversion |

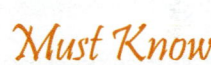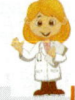

Must Know

In the clinical setting, the distinction between narrow and wide complex tachycardia (supraventricular vs. ventricular) is fundamental since they are treated differently.

Paroxysmal Supraventricular Tachycardia (PSVT)

- SVT that **starts or ends very suddenly** is called PSVT.
- PSVT is a rapid rhythm that starts and stops suddenly.
- For accurate interpretation, the beginning or end of the PSVT must be seen.
- PSVT, a relatively common arrhythmia, arises from reentry in dual pathways within the AV node or through accessory pathways in patients with the Wolff–Parkinson–White syndrome.

Key Features

- PSVT stands for paroxysmal (which means sudden onset), supraventricular (coming from above the ventricles) tachycardia (rate greater than 100).
- The only difference between PSVT and SVT is that the onset of the PSVT can be seen. In PATs, the origin of the rapid beats is clearly in the atria whereas in PSVTs and SVTs, a strict determination cannot be made.
- Ectopic focus may be present anywhere above the bifurcation of the bundle of His.
- Impulse arise and recycle repeatedly in the AV node because of areas of unidirectional block in the Purkinje fibers.
- In PSVT, re-excitation of the atria may occur when there is a one way block.
- PSVT, as the name implies, is paroxysmal, but occasionally re-entrant SVT may be persistent or permanent, a pattern that occurs less often in adults

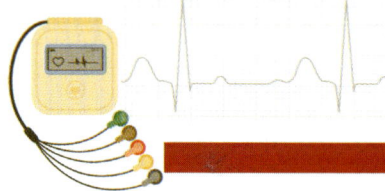

than in children, in whom the persistent arrhythmia may produce reversible cardiomyopathy.

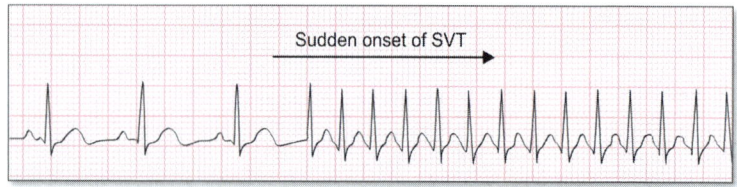

Sudden onset of SVT

Fig. 7.12 ECG showing paroxysmal supraventricular tachycardia (PSVT)

Note: Sudden change in rate is a characteristic feature of PSVT.

Characteristics of paroxysmal supraventricular tachycardia have been described in Table 7.8.

Table 7.8 Charceristics of paroxysmal supraventricular tachycardia (PSVT)

ECG Characteristics (Fig. 7.12)	**Rhythm**	Regular
	Atrial rate	Variable
	Ventricular rate	150–250 bpm
	P wave	Frequently buried in preceding T waves and difficult to see
	PR interval	Usually not possible to measure
	QRS	Normal (0.06–0.10 sec) but may be wide if abnormally conducted through ventricles
	T wave	Variable
	QT interval	Varies from normal to less than normal
Causes	• Over exertion • Emotional stress	• Deep inspiration • RHD, CAD, COPD and CHF
Signs and Symptoms	• Prolonged episode and heart rate greater than 180 beats/min • Decreased cardiac output-hypotension, dyspnea & angina • Light headedness, palpitations • Anxious and uncomfortable	
Management	**Medical**	• Vagal stimulation such as carotid massage (which may abort the attack) (Fig. 7.13). • IV adenosine • IV Verapamil- 5-10 mg • Beta blockers • Cardio version • Calcium channel blockers
	Nursing	Nursing management is same as for SVT

Abbreviations: RHD, rheumatic heart disease, CAD, coronary artery disease; COPD, chronic obstructive pulmonary disease; CHF, congestive heart failure; IV, intravenous; SVT, supraventricular tachycardia.

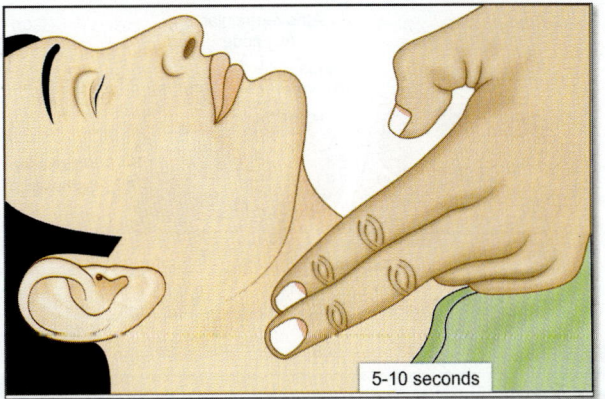

5-10 seconds

Fig. 7.13 Carotid massage

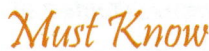

Must Know

- It is the most frequent regular tachyarrhythmia in adults, and atrioventricular nodal re-entry is the more common mechanism.
- When PSVT first appears in relatively young subjects, the re-entry is more often sustained in accessory pathways. Re-entry in accessory pathways is more common in men and intranodal re-entry in women.
- Most of the patients with PSVT have no structural heart disease.

Wolff-Parkinson-White (WPW) Syndrome

In WPW, an **accessory conduction pathway** is present between the atria and the ventricles. Electrical impulses are rapidly conducted to the ventricles. These rapid impulses create a slurring of the initial portion of the QRS called the delta wave.

WPW syndrome is a **congenital condition** involving abnormal conductive cardiac tissue between atria and ventricles. Accessory conduction pathway is provided by that tissue forming reentrant tachycardia circuit which leads to pre-excitation of the ventricles (Figs 7.14A and B).

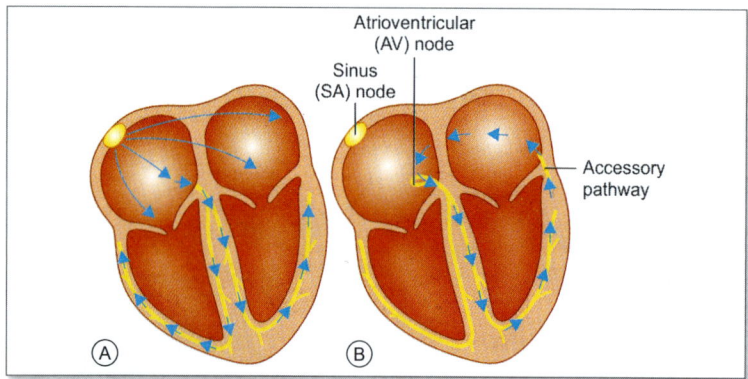

Figs 7.14A and B Wolff-Parkinson-White (WPW) Syndrome: (A) Normal electrical pathways; (B) Abnormal electrical pathway in Wolff-Parkinson-White syndrome

Key Features (Table 7.9)

- WPW may be described as type A, B or C.
  - **Type A:** The delta waves are predominantly upright in all of the precordial leads.
  - **Type B:** The delta waves are predominantly negative in leads V1-V3 and predominantly positive in leads V4-V6. It can be mistaken for left bundle branch block or left ventricular hypertrophy with strain.
  - **Type C:** The delta waves are upright in leads V1-V4 but negative in leads V5-V6.

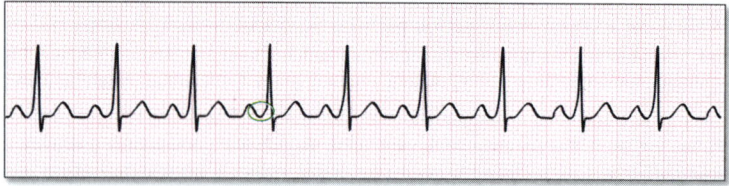

Fig. 7.15 ECG showing Wolff-Parkinson-White (WPW) Syndrome

Characteristics of WPW syndrome have been described in Table 7.9.

Table 7.9 Characteristics of Wolff-Parkinson-White (WPW) Syndrome

ECG Characteristics (Fig. 7.15)	**Rhythm**	Regular unless atrial fibrillation present
	Atrial rate	Normal
	Ventricular rate	Normal
	P wave	Normal
	PR interval	Short PR interval (less than 0.10 second)
	QRS	• Broad QRS (greater than 0.10 second) • A slurred upstroke to the QRS complex (the delta wave)
	T wave	ST Segment and T wave discordant changes – i.e. in the opposite direction to the major component of the QRS complex
Causes		Congenital heart abnormality such as Ebstein anomaly and may also run in family.
Signs and Symptoms		• Palpitations • Dizziness • Dyspnea • Anxiety • Syncope • Rarely, cardiac arrest (sudden death) • Some people have WPW without any symptoms at all.
Management	**Medical**	• In the absence of symptoms, treatment is not required. • Treated if tachyarrhythmias, such as atrial fibrillation and atrial flutter, occur. • First, electrophysiology studies are done to determine the location of the conduction pathway and evaluate specific treatments. • Radiofrequency ablation may be used with resistant tachyarrhythmia (Fig. 7.16). • Instruct the patients to perform vagal maneuvers to help slow down a rapid heartbeat when it occurs.
	Nursing	• Remember that atrial fibrillation with a wide QRS complex may indicate Wolff-Parkinson-White (WPW) syndrome; in such cases, use of AV node blocking drugs may be fatal. • Do not give digoxin or non-dihydropyridine calcium channel blockers (e.g. verapamil, diltiazem) to patients with atrial fibrillation and WPW because these drugs may trigger ventricular fibrillation.

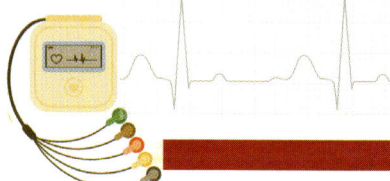

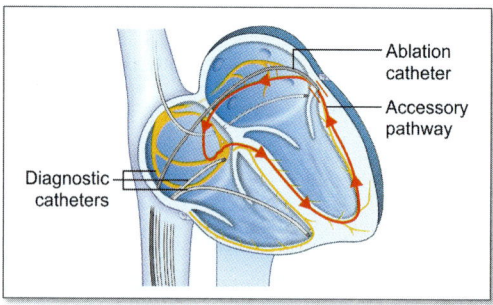

Fig. 7.16 Radio frequency ablation

Must Know

- First described in 1930 by Louis Wolff, John Parkinson and Paul Dudley White.
- Wolff-Parkinson-White (WPW) Syndrome is a combination of the presence of a congenital accessory pathway and episodes of tachyarrhythmia.
- In WPW, the accessory pathway is often referred to as the Bundle of Kent, or atrioventricular bypass tract.
- A pseudo-infarction pattern can be seen in up to 70% of patients – due to negatively deflected delta waves in the inferior/anterior leads ("pseudo-Q waves"), or as a prominent R wave in V1-3 (mimicking posterior infarction) Figure 7.17.

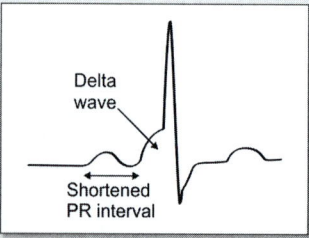

Fig. 7.17 Delta wave in WPW Syndrome

NURSING PROCESS APPLIED FOR THE PATIENT HAVING ATRIAL ARRHYTHMIAS

Decreased cardiac output

Nursing Assessment

Hypotension, cool and clammy skin, rapid and irregular pulse.

Nursing Diagnosis

Decreased cardiac output related to loss of atrial mechanical activity as evidenced by hypotension, cool and clammy skin.

Planning

To maintain cardiac output

Nursing Interventions

- Assess vital signs
- Monitor skin changes color, moisture, temperature and capillary refill time
- Obtain 12 lead ECG and interpret the findings
- Maintain airway, breathing and circulation on priority basis
- Administer medications such as beta-blockers, calcium, amiodarone and digitalis as prescribed by the physician.
- Cardioversion may be the initial treatment of choice if the patient is haemodynamically unstable
- Prepare for cardioversion as indicated.
- If an emergency cardioversion is required for haemodynamic compromise it is important to explain the procedure and reassure the patient.

Evaluation

Expected patient outcome may include maintenance of cardiac output.

Risk for Thromboembolism

Nursing Assessment

Altered mental status, confusion, and weak peripheral pulses

Nursing Diagnosis

Risk for thromboembolism related to atrial fibrillation.

Planning

To prevent the episodes of thromboembolism.

Nursing Interventions

- Monitor cardiac rhythm as indicated.
- Promote bed rest with head of the bed elevated to 45°.
- Monitor blood pressure, apical pulse and peripheral pulses.

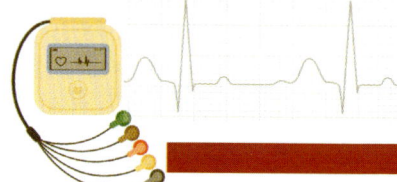

- Observe patient for restlessness, agitation, confusion and (late stages) lethargy
- Monitor mental status changes.
- Monitor patient intake, output and maintain chart every hour
- Assess peripheral pulses
- Administer anticoagulants as prescribed.
- For assessing the early symptoms of stroke (one of the common thromboembolic episode with atrial fibrillation) teach family members about FAST acronym which stands for Facial drooping, Arm weakness, Speech difficulties and Time to call emergency services.

Evaluation

Expected patient outcome may include prevention from thromboembolic episodes.

Risk for Bleeding

Nursing Assessment

- Use of anticoagulants
- Altered coagulation status

Nursing Diagnosis

Risk for bleeding related to use of anticoagulants.

Planning

To prevent bleeding.

Nursing Interventions

- Monitor patients vital signs, especially BP and HR as hypotension and tachycardia are initial compensatory mechanisms usually noted with bleeding.
- Assess skin and mucous membranes for signs of petechiae, bruising, hematoma formation or oozing of blood.
- Review laboratory results for coagulation status as appropriate.
- Advice the patient to take bleeding precautions as given below:
  - Use a soft bristled toothbrush. Avoid the use of dental floss and toothpicks.
  - Avoid rectal suppositories, thermometers, enemas, vaginal douches and tampoons.
  - Limit straining with bowel movements, forceful nose blowing, coughing and sneezing.
  - Be careful when using sharp objects like scissors and knives. Use an electric razor for shaving (not razor blades).

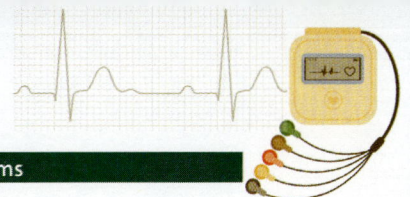

- Tell the female patient to inform the health care provider when there is an increase in menstrual bleeding as indicated by an increase in the number of sanitary pads used.
- Educate the patient and family members about signs of bleeding that need to be reported to a health care provider.

Evaluation

Expected patient outcome may include gaining confidence to follow bleeding precautions.

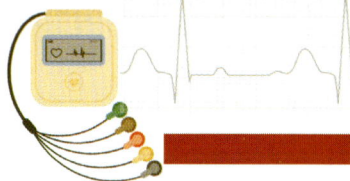

 Practice Questions

1. **Most common arrhythmia present among ICU patients is:**
   a. Atrial flutter
   b. Atrial fibrillation
   c. Paroxysmal supraventricular tachycardia
   d. WPW syndrome

2. **A patient develops sudden palpitations with heart rate of 150 beats/min and the rhythm is regular. What can be the cause?**
   a. Atrial flutter
   b. Ventricular tachycardia
   c. Paroxysmal supraventricular tachycardia
   d. Supra ventricular tachycardia

3. **Radiofrequency ablation is done for:**
   a. Atrial tachycardia
   b. Ventricular tachycardia
   c. Paroxysmal supraventricular tachycardia
   d. WPW syndrome

4. **Most common benign cardiac rhythm is:**
   a. Premature atrial complex
   b. Premature ventricular complex
   c. Atrial fibrillation
   d. Ventricular tachycardia

5. **Identify the rhythm:**

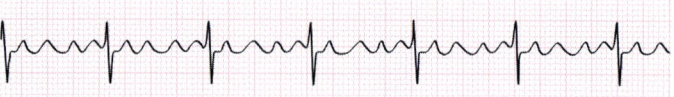

6. **Identify the rhythm:**

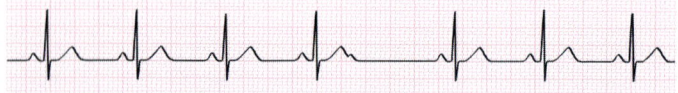

7. **Identify the rhythm:**

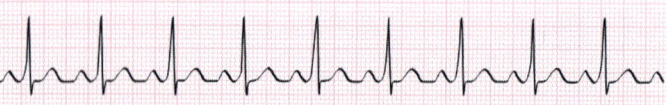

8. **Identify the rhythm:**

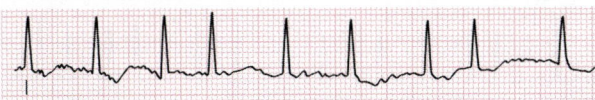

9. **Identify the rhythm:**

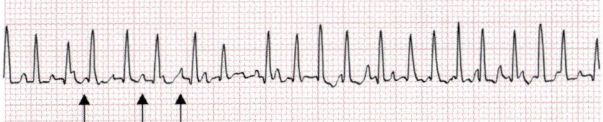

10. **All are true about WPW syndrome except:**
    a. Can occur in a normal heart
    b. More common in females
    c. Delta wave in ECG
    d. Short PR interval

11. **Which of the following arrhythmia is most commonly associated with alcohol binge in alcoholics:**
    a. Ventricular fibrillation
    b. Atrial fibrillation
    c. Atrial flutter
    d. Premature ventricular contraction

12. **Identify the rhythm:**

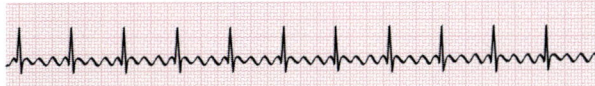

13. **Identify the rhythm:**

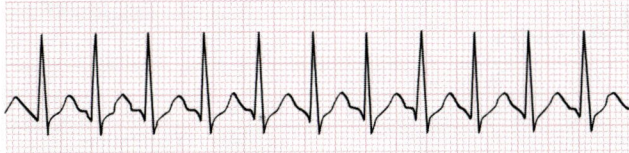

14. **Identify the rhythm:**

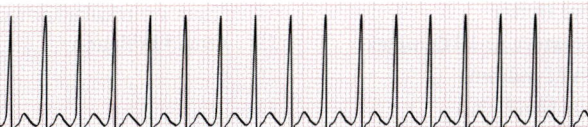

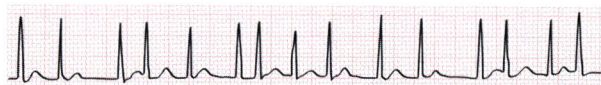

15. Identify the rhythm:

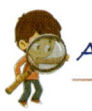

16. All of the following are true about atrial fibrillation except:
   a. Risk of thromboembolism
   b. Digoxin for treatment
   c. Cardioversion followed by anticoagulation
   d. Ectopic originating in pulmonary veins

17. An 18-year-old boy is asymptomatic. On ECG, he has a short PR interval with delta waves. Which of the following is not routinely required for this patient.
   a. Holter monitoring
   b. Reassurance
   c. Treadmill test
   d. Beta blocker

Answers

1.	b	10.	b
2.	c	11.	Atrial fibrillation
3.	d	12.	Atrial Flutter
4.	a	13.	Supra ventricular tachycardia
5.	Atrial Flutter	14.	Supra ventricular tachycardia
6.	Premature Atrial Complex	15.	Atrial fibrillation
7.	WPW Syndrome	16.	c
8.	Atrial fibrillation	17.	c
9.	Multifocal Atrial tachycardia		

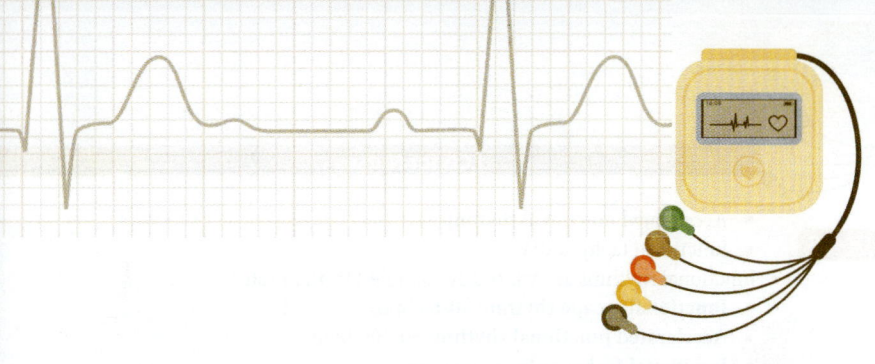

Junctional Rhythms

Chapter 8

INTRODUCTION

- The sinoatrial (SA) node is the normal origin of the electrical impulse for a heartbeat. When the SA node cannot perform this role, the atrioventricular (AV) node may take-over pace making. When this occurs, the electrocardiogram (ECG) will likely have distinctive waveform features that reveal important aspects of these junctional rhythms.
- Arrhythmias that arise in automatic tissues of the AV node or bundle of His are called junctional arrhythmias because the tissues involved lie in the region where the atria and ventricles join (Fig. 8.1).

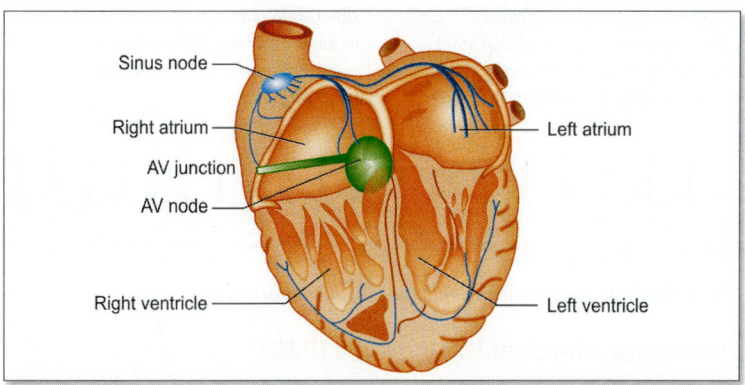

Fig. 8.1 AV Junction which is made up of the AV node and the AV bundle

CLASSIFICATION OF JUNCTIONAL ARRHYTHMIAS

- Broadly junctional arrhythmias can be divided into following main sub classifications (Table 8.1):
  - Premature junctional contraction (PJC)
  - Junctional escape rhythm

- Accelerated junctional rhythm
- Junctional tachycardia
- Junctional rhythms are arbitrarily classified by their rate:
  - **Junctional escape rhythm:** 40-60 bpm
  - **Accelerated junctional rhythm:** 60-100 bpm
  - **Junctional tachycardia:**> 100 bpm
- They may also be classified by etiology:
  - **Automatic junctional rhythms** (AJR) = Due to enhanced automaticity in AV nodal cells
  - **Re-entrant junctional rhythms** (AVNRT) = Due to re-entrant loop involving AV node

Table 8.1 Classification of junctional rhythm

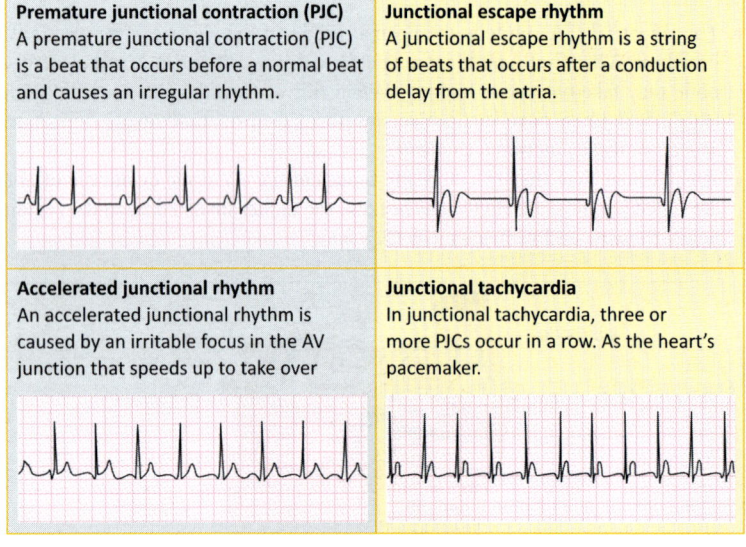

Premature junctional contraction (PJC) A premature junctional contraction (PJC) is a beat that occurs before a normal beat and causes an irregular rhythm.	**Junctional escape rhythm** A junctional escape rhythm is a string of beats that occurs after a conduction delay from the atria.
Accelerated junctional rhythm An accelerated junctional rhythm is caused by an irritable focus in the AV junction that speeds up to take over	**Junctional tachycardia** In junctional tachycardia, three or more PJCs occur in a row. As the heart's pacemaker.

These rhythms are described separately, in subsequent pages.

Premature Junctional Complexes (PJCs)

A PJC is a beat that occurs before a normal beat and causes an irregular rhythm.

Key Feature

This ectopic beat occurs when an irritable location within the AV junction acts as a pacemaker and fires either prematurely or out of sequence.

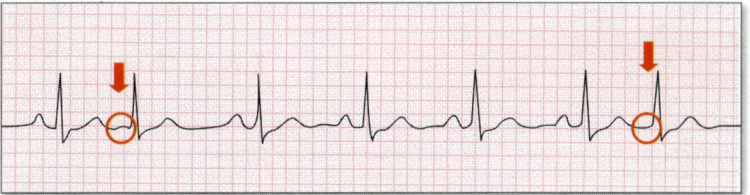

Fig. 8.2 ECG showing premature junctional complex

Note: Note the hidden P wave.

Characteristics of premature junctional complex have been described in Table 8.2.

Table 8.2 Characteristics of premature junctional complex

ECG Characteristics (Fig. 8.2)	**Rhythm**	Irregular atrial and ventricular rhythms
	Atrial rate	100 beats/minute
	Ventricular rate	100 beats/minute
	P wave	Inverted or hidden. May fall before, during, or after the QRS complex with PJC; otherwise normal configuration
	PR interval	If P wave comes before the QRS complex, the PR interval is less than 0.12 second.
	QRS	Normal
	T wave	Normal
	QT interval	Normal
Causes	• Toxic levels of digoxin (level greater than 2.5 ng/ml) • Excessive caffeine intake • Inferior wall myocardial infarction (MI) • Rheumatic heart disease • Hypoxia • Heart failure, or swelling of the AV junction after heart surgery	
Signs and Symptoms	• Asymptomatic initially • Palpitations or a feeling of quickening in the chest • Irregular pulse • If the PJCs are frequent enough, the patient may have hypotension from a transient decrease in cardiac output	
Management	**Medical**	• PJCs usually don't require treatment unless symptoms occur. • Treatment of the underlying cause. • If digoxin toxicity is the culprit, the medication should be discontinued. • Monitor the patient for hemodynamic instability.
	Nursing	• Monitor serum level of digoxin if the patient is taking digoxin. • If ectopic beats are frequent, the patient should decrease or eliminate his/her caffeine intake.

Must Know

As with all beats produced by the AV junction, the atria are depolarized in retrograde fashion, causing an inverted P wave. The ventricles are depolarized normally.

Junctional Escape Rhythm

A junctional escape rhythm is a string of beats that occurs after a conduction delay from the atria.

Key Features

- AV junction can take over as the heart's pacemaker if higher pacemaker sites slow down or fail to fire or conduct. The junctional escape beat is an example of this compensatory mechanism.
- Junctional escape beats prevent ventricular standstill, therefore they should never be suppressed.

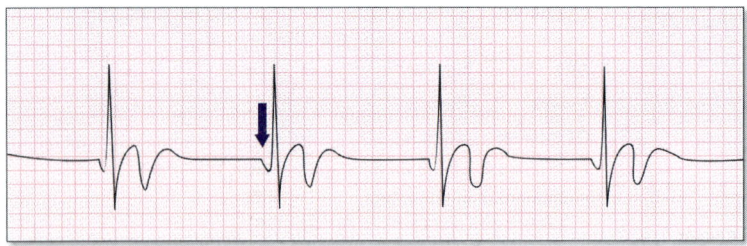

Fig. 8.3 ECG showing junctional escape rhythm

Characteristics of junctional escape rhythm have been described in Table 8.3.

Table 8.3 Characteristics of junctional escape rhythm

	Rhythm	Regular
	Atrial rate	40-60 beats/minute
	Ventricular rate	40-60 beats/minute
ECG Characteristics (Fig. 8.3)	**P wave**	Inverted and preceding each QRS complex
	PR interval	0.10 second
	QRS	Normal
	T wave	Normal
	QT interval	Normal

Contd...

Causes	• Sick Sinus Syndrome • Vagal Stimulation • Digoxin Toxicity • Inferior Wall MI • Rheumatic Heart Disease.	
Signs and Symptoms	• Slow, regular pulse rate of 40 to 60 beats/minute. • May be asymptomatic. • If pulse rates less than 60 beats/minute may lead to inadequate cardiac output, causing hypotension, syncope, or decreased urine output.	
Management	Medical	• Correcting the underlying cause; such as digoxin may be withheld. • Atropine • Temporary or permanent pacemaker if the patient is symptomatic
	Nursing	• Monitor patient's serum digoxin and electrolyte levels. • Observe for signs of decreased cardiac output, such as hypotension, syncope, or decreased urine output. • If the patient is hypotensive, lower the head of his bed as far as he can tolerate it. • Keep atropine at the bedside. • Discontinue digoxin if indicated.

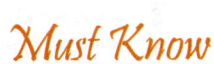 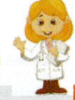

Must Know

• Junctional escape beats may occur in healthy children during sleep.
• They may also occur in healthy athletic adults.

Accelerated Junctional Rhythm

An accelerated junctional rhythm is caused by an irritable focus in the AV junction that speeds up to take over as the heart's pacemaker.

Key Features

• The atria are depolarized by means of retrograde conduction, and the ventricles are depolarized normally.
• The accelerated rate is usually between 60 and 100 beats/minute

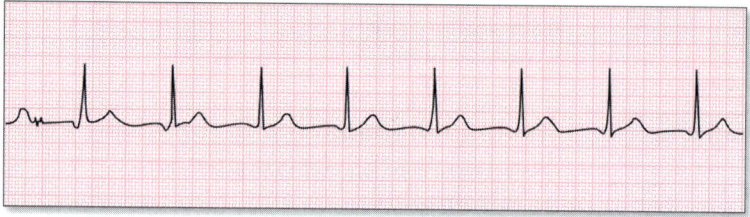

ECG showing accelerated junctional rhythm

Characteristics of accelerated junctional rhythm have been described in Table 8.4.

Table 8.4 Characteristics of accelerated junctional rhythm

ECG Characteristics (Fig. 8.4)	**Rhythm**	Regular
	Atrial rate	60 to 100 beats/minute.
	Ventricular rate	60 to 100 beats/minute.
	P wave	Inverted in leads II, III, and aVF and will occur before or after the QRS complex or be hidden in it.
	PR interval	If the P wave comes before the QRS complex, the PR interval will be less than 0.12 second.
	QRS	Normal
	T wave	Normal
	QT interval	Normal
Causes		• Digoxin toxicity • Hypokalaemia • Inferior or posterior wall myocardial infarction (MI) • Rheumatic heart disease • Valvular heart disease.
Signs and Symptoms		• The patient may be asymptomatic because accelerated junctional rhythm has the same rate as sinus rhythm. • If cardiac output is low, the patient may become dizzy, hypotensive, and confused and have weak peripheral pulses.
Management	**Medical**	• Correcting the underlying cause. • Temporary pacing may be necessary if the patient is symptomatic.
	Nursing	• Observe the patient to see how well he tolerates this arrhythmia. • Monitor serum digoxin level of patient, and withhold digoxin dose as instructed • Assess potassium and other electrolyte levels and administer supplements as ordered. • Monitor vital signs for hemodynamic instability; and observe for signs of decreased cardiac output.

Must Know

Accelerated junctional rhythm arises when there is increased automaticity in the AV node coupled with decreased automaticity in the sinus node.

Junctional Tachycardia

In junctional tachycardia, three or more PJCs occur in a row. This supra ventricular tachycardia occurs when an irritable focus from the AV junction has enhanced automaticity, overriding the SA node to function as the heart's pacemaker.

Key Feature

In this arrhythmia, the atria are depolarized by means of retrograde conduction, and conduction through the ventricles is normal.

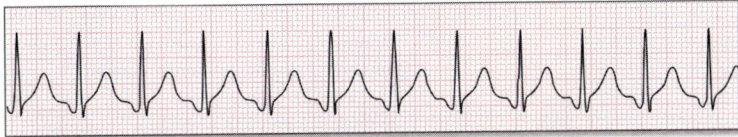

Fig. 8.5 ECG showing junctional tachycardia

Characteristics of junctional tachycardia have been described in Table 8.5.

Table 8.5 Characteristics of junctional tachycardia

ECG Characteristics (Fig. 8.5)	**Rhythm**	Regular
	Atrial rate	100 to 200 beats/minute
	Ventricular rate	100 to 200 beats/minute
	P wave	Inverted; follows QRS complex in leads II, III, and aVF
	PR interval	Immeasurable
	QRS	Normal
	T wave	Normal
	QT interval	Normal
Causes	• Digoxin toxicity (most common cause), which can be enhanced by hypokalemia • Inferior or posterior wall myocardial infarction (MI) or ischemia • Congenital heart disease in children • Swelling of the AV junction after heart surgery	

Contd...

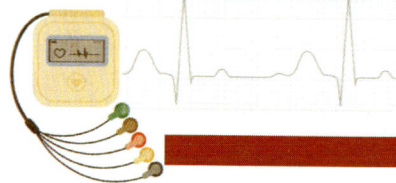

Signs and Symptoms	• Patients with rapid heart rates may have decreased cardiac output and hemodynamic instability. • The pulse will be rapid, and dizziness, low blood pressure, and other signs of decreased cardiac output may be present.	
Management	Medical	• The underlying cause should be treated. • If the cause is digoxin toxicity, the digoxin should be discontinued. • Vagal maneuvers and medications such as verapamil may slow the heart rate for the symptomatic patient. • If the patient recently had an MI or heart surgery, he may need a temporary pacemaker to reset the heart's rhythm. • A child with a permanent arrhythmia may be resistant to drug therapy and require surgery. • The patient with recurrent junctional tachycardia may be treated with ablation therapy, followed by permanent pacemaker insertion.
	Nursing	• Monitor patients with junctional tachycardia for signs of decreased cardiac output • Check serum digoxin and potassium levels and administer potassium supplements, as ordered. • If symptoms are severe and digoxin is the culprit, then administer digoxin immune fab, a digoxin-binding drug as prescribed.

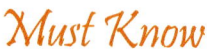

Must Know

• Junctional tachycardia is not a reentrant SVT. It arises from the AV junction including Bundle of His.
• ECG characteristics are similar to accelerated junctional rhythm except for the rate.

NURSING PROCESS APPLIED FOR THE PATIENT HAVING JUNCTIONAL ARRHYTHMIAS

Decreased Cardiac Output

Nursing Assessment

Dizziness, hypotension and weak peripheral pulses.

Nursing Diagnosis

Decreased cardiac output related to disease condition as evidenced by dizziness, hypotension and weak peripheral pulses.

Planning

To maintain the normal cardiac output

Nursing Interventions

- Monitor vital signs for hemodynamic instability; and observe for signs of decreased cardiac output.
- Obtain 12 lead ECG and interpret the findings.
- Check serum digoxin and potassium levels.
- Administer the medications as prescribed.
- If symptoms are severe and digoxin is the culprit, then administer digoxin immune fab, a digoxin-binding drug as prescribed and for hypokalemia (if present), administer potassium supplements, as instructed.
- May need to prepare for ablation therapy.
- Prepare for permanent pacemaker insertion as instructed and provide detailed patient explanation for the same.

Evaluation

Expected patient outcome may include maintenance of normal cardiac output.

Fatigue

Nursing Assessment

Decreased performance, failure to maintain usual routines, lethargic or sluggish, tired.

Nursing Diagnosis

Fatigue secondary to decreased cardiac output as evidenced by lethargy, tiredness and decreased performance.

Planning

- Ability to perform activities of daily living properly.
- To demonstrate energy saving techniques which will help in reducing fatigue.

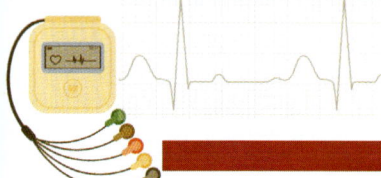

Nursing Interventions

- Evaluate the patient's description of fatigue: severity, changes in severity over time, aggregating factors or alleviating factors.
- Assess the patient's ability to perform ADLs.
- Restrict environmental stimuli, especially during planned times for rest and sleep.
- Aid the patient with developing a schedule for daily activity and rest. Emphasize the importance of frequent rest periods.
- Teach energy conservation methods.
- Encourage an exercise conditioning program as appropriate.
- Encourage verbalization of feelings about the impact of fatigue.
- Set practical activity goals with patient.
- Aid the patient develops habits to promote effective rest/sleep patterns.
- As the reason for fatigue is decreased cardiac output associated with junctional arrhythmias, administer antiarrhythmics as prescribed.
- Monitor the patient closely to assess the impact of interventions performed.

Evaluation

Expected patient outcome may include ability to perform activities of daily living by him/her.

Practice Questions

1. **Accelerated junctional rhythm is characterized by:**
   a. Rate below 40 beats/min   b. Rate between 40-60 beats/min
   c. Rate of 60-100 beats/min   d. Rate above 100 beats/min

2. **Junctional escape rhythm is characterized by:**
   a. Rate below 40 beats/min   b. Rate between 40-60 beats/min
   c. Rate of 60-100 beats/min   d. Rate above 100 beats/min

3. **Identify the rhythm:**

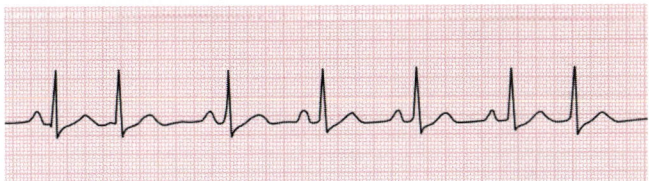

4. **Identify the rhythm:**

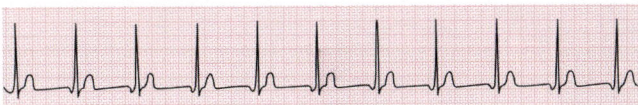

5. **Identify the rhythm:**

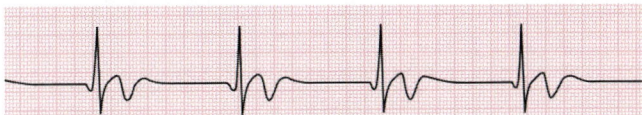

6. **Junctional bradycardia is characterized by:**
   a. Rate below 40 beats/min   b. Rate between 40-60 beats/min
   c. Rate of 60-100 beats/min   d. Rate above 100 beats/min

7. **Identify the rhythm:**

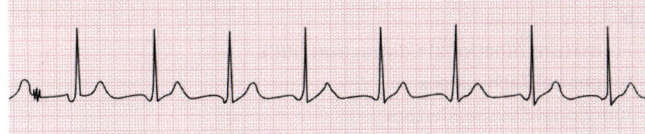

8. **Junctional tachycardia is characterized by:**
   a. Rate below 40 beats/min   b. Rate between 40-60 beats/min
   c. Rate of 60-100 beats/min   d. Rate above 100 beats/min

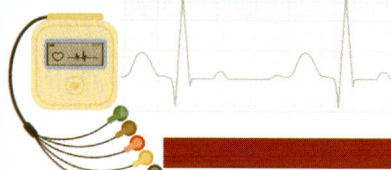

9. The monitor shows regular QRS complexes with a constant QRS width of 0.08 seconds. The ventricular rate is 68 b/min and no P waves are visible. This rhythm is:
   a. Idioventricular rhythm
   b. Junctional bradycardia
   c. Accelerated Junctional Rhythm
   d. Atrial fibrillation

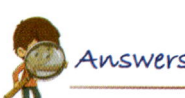

Answers

1. c
2. b
3. Premature Junctional Contraction (PJC)
4. Junctional Tachycardia
5. Junctional Escape Rhythm
6. a
7. Accelerated Junctional Rhythm
8. d
9. c

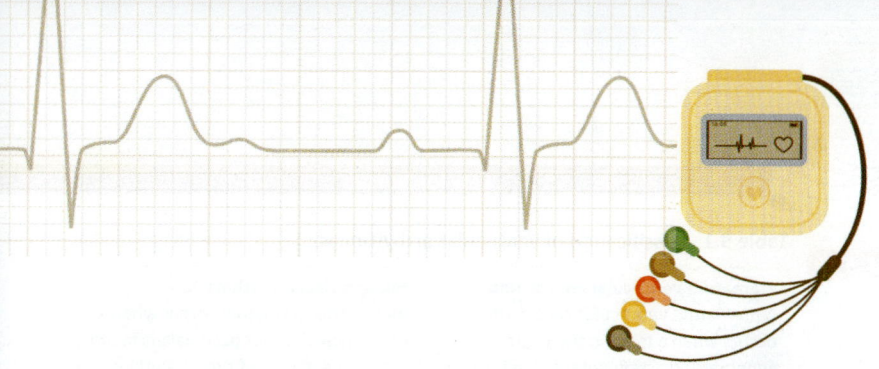

Ventricular Arrhythmias

Chapter **9**

INTRODUCTION

- Failure of the sinoatrial (SA) node and the atrioventricular (AV) junctional tissues to generate an impulse leads to activation of the ventricles as pacemaker of the heart. Ventricular arrhythmias arise from the ventricles and are characterized by abnormally wide and bizarre QRS complexes, fast heart rates and typically absence of P waves. There is an absence of P waves because there is no atrial activity or depolarization
- Ventricular arrhythmias are wide complex rhythms that may be regular or irregular. These may be normal rate, bradycardia or tachycardia and may occur as single beats or sustained. Some ventricular arrhythmias may present as sudden cardiac arrest.
- Wide complexes occur because rhythm comes from the ventricles and do not use the normal ventricular conduction system; action potentials need to travel from one myocyte to another, which is much slower, creating a wide QRS complex.

CLASSIFICATION OF VENTRICULAR ARRHYTHMIAS (TABLE 9.1)

Broadly ventricular arrhythmias can be divided into following main sub classifications:

- Premature ventricular contraction (PVC)
- Idioventricular rhythms
- Ventricular tachycardia
- Ventricular fibrillation (VFib)
- Pulseless electrical activity
- Agonal rhythm
- Asystole

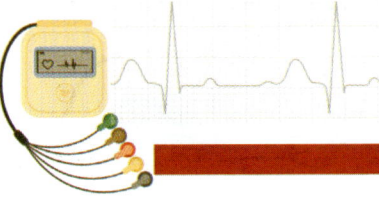

Table 9.1 Classification of ventricular arrhythmias

Premature ventricular contraction A premature ventricular contraction occurs when a focus in the ventricle generates an action potential before the next scheduled sinoatrial nodal action potential. 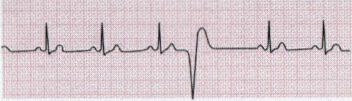	**Idioventricular rhythms** Idioventricular rhythms occur when all of the heart's other pacemakers fail to function and cells of the His Purkinje system act as heart's pacemaker to generate electrical impulses. 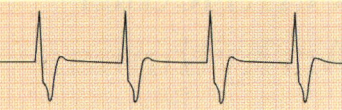
Ventricular tachycardia Ventricular tachycardia (V-tach) is a rhythm with a rapid recurrence of premature ventricular contractions with no normal beats in between. 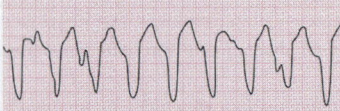	**Ventricular fibrillation (V-Fib)** Occurs as a result of multiple weak ectopic foci in the ventricles characterized by no coordinated atrial or ventricular contraction, electrical impulses initiated by multiple ventricular sites and impulses are not transmitted through normal conduction pathway. 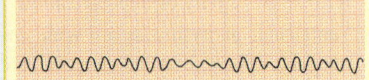
Pulseless electrical activity Pulseless electrical activity (PEA) encompasses a heterogenous group of rhythms that are organized or semi organized but lack a palpable pulse. 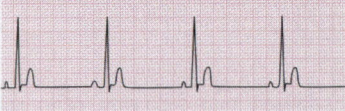	**Agonal rhythm** Agonal rhythm is when the idioventricular rhythm is 20 beats or less per minute 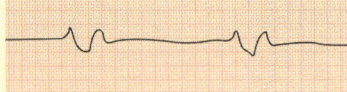
Asystole Asystole is a dire form of cardiac arrest in which the heart stops beating and there is no electrical activity in the heart. As a result, the heart is at a total standstill. 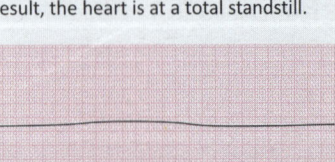	

These rhythms are described separately, in subsequent pages.

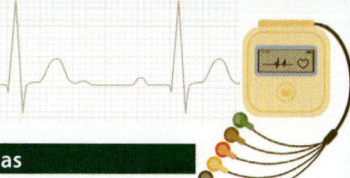

Premature Ventricular Contraction (Fig. 9.1)

Premature ventricular contraction is a relatively common event where the heartbeat is initiated by Purkinje fibers in the ventricles rather than by the SA node, the normal heartbeat initiator.

It is also known as a premature ventricular complex, ventricular premature contraction (VPC), ventricular premature beat (VPB), or ventricular extrasystole (VES).

Early ventricular contraction results from increased irritability of ventricles caused by an ectopic cardiac pacemaker located in ventricle.

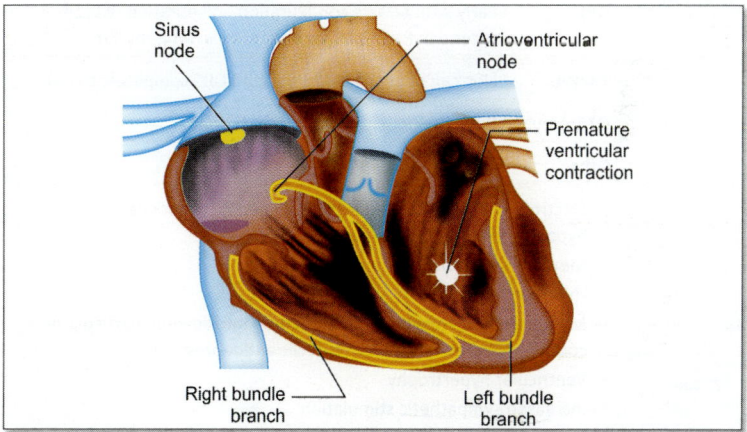

Fig. 9.1 Diagrammatic representation of premature ventricular contraction

Key Features

- Originating ectopic focus in the ventricles.
- Premature occurrence of a QRS complex which is wide and distorted in shape
- Although a PVC can be a sign of decreased oxygenation to the heart muscle, often PVCs are benign and may even be found in otherwise healthy hearts.
- Patients may sense the occurrence of PVCs as skipped beats. Because the ventricles are only partially filled, the PVC frequently does not generate a pulse.
- The pause following a PVC may be compensatory or non–compensatory.

Characteristics of premature ventricular complex have been given Table 9.2.

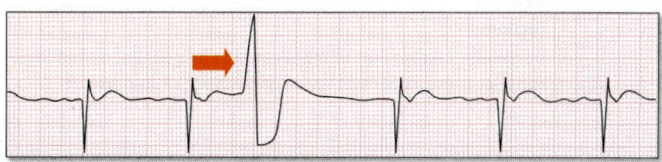

Fig. 9.2 ECG showing premature ventricular complex

Table 9.2 Characteristics of premature ventricular complex

ECG Characteristics (Fig. 9.2)	**Rhythm**	Irregular
	Atrial rate	Usually normal
	Ventricular rate	Usually normal (depends on the underlying rhythm)
	P wave	Absent with PVC, but present with other QRS complexes
	PR interval	0.12 second in underlying rhythm
	QRS	Early with bizarre configuration and duration of 0.14 second in PVC; 0.08 second in underlying rhythm
	T wave	Normal; opposite direction from QRS complex with PVC
	QT interval	0.28 second with under lying rhythm
	Other	Compensatory pause after PVC
Causes		• Electrolyte imbalances, such as hypokalemia, hyperkalemia, hypomagnaesemia, and hypocalcaemia • Metabolic acidosis • Hypoxia • Myocardial ischemia and infarction drug intoxication, particularly cocaine, amphetamines, and tricyclic antidepressants • Ventricular hypertrophy • Increased sympathetic stimulation • Myocarditis • Cardiomyopathy • Heart failure • Caffeine or alcohol ingestion • Proarrhythmic effects of some antiarrhythmics • Tobacco use.
Signs and Symptoms		• On palpation, much weaker pulse wave after the premature beat and a longer-than-normal pause between pulse waves. At times, absence of any pulse after the PVC. • On Auscultation, an abnormally early heart sound and a diminished amplitude with each premature beat • Palpitations, hypotension or syncope with frequent PVCs. • Dyspnea • Dizziness • Decreased cardiac output manifested as fatigue, decreased level of consciousness, cool peripheries, increased JVP, hypoxemia

Contd...

Manage-ment	Medical	• If the patient is asymptomatic, the arrhythmia probably won't require treatment. • If he has symptoms or a dangerous form of PVCs, the type of treatment depends on the cause of the problem. • Treatment consists of procainamide (Procan), amiodarone (Cordarone), or lidocaine I.V. (first line drug) • Potassium chloride may be given I.V. to correct hypokalaemia, and magnesium sulfate I.V. may be given to correct hypomagnaesemia. • O_2 administration for hypoxia • Radiofrequency catheter ablation treatment • Implantable cardioverter-defibrillator • Other treatments may be aimed at adjusting drug therapy or correcting acidosis, hypothermia, or hypoxia.
	Nursing	• Patients who have recently developed PVCs need prompt assessment, especially if they have underlying heart disease or complex medical problems. • Frequently stressed individuals should consider therapy, or joining a support group. • Those with chronic PVCs should be observed closely for the development of more frequent PVCs or more dangerous PVC patterns. • Until an effective treatment is begun, a patient with PVCs accompanied by serious symptoms should have continuous ECG monitoring and ambulate only with assistance. • If the patient is discharged from the health care facility on antiarrhythmic drugs, family members should know how to contact the emergency medical service (EMS) and how to perform cardiopulmonary resuscitation (CPR).

Types of PVCs

• **Bigeminy, Trigeminy and Quadrigeminy:** PVCs that occur every other beat (bigeminy) or every third beat (trigeminy) or every fourth beat (quadrigeminy) may indicate increased ventricular irritability.

Bigeminy

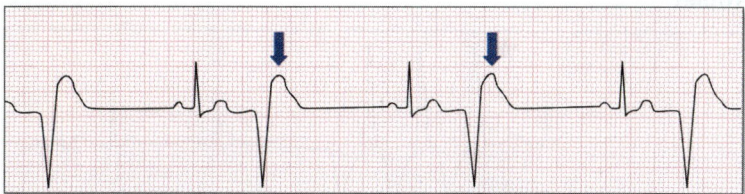

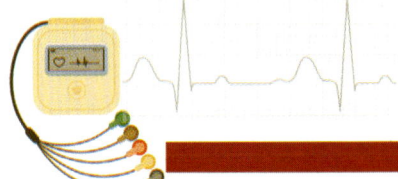

Trigeminy

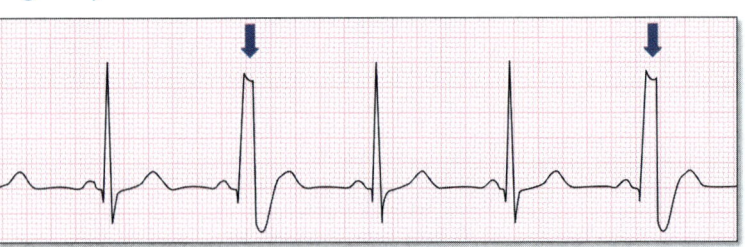

Quadrigeminy

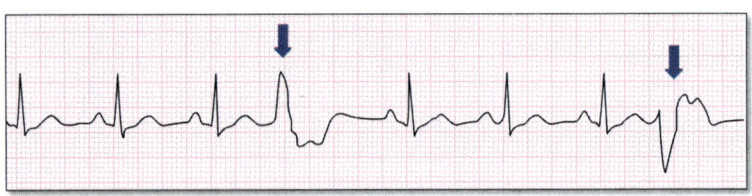

Paired PVCs

Two PVCs in a row are called a pair, or couplet. A pair can produce ventricular tachycardia because the second depolarization usually meets refractory tissue. **A salvo—three or more PVCs in a row—is considered a run of ventricular tachycardia.**

Couplet

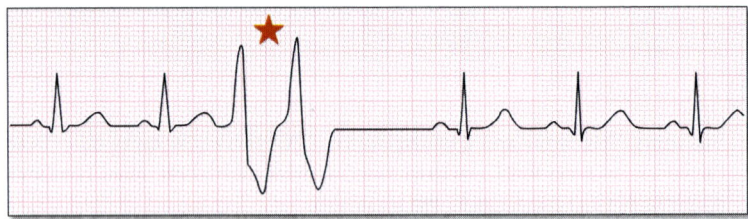

Triplet

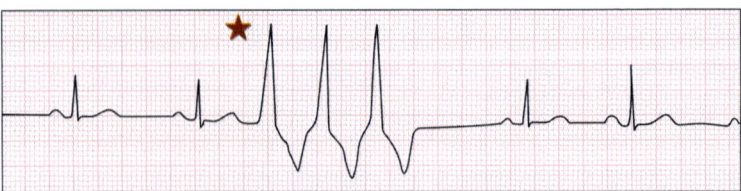

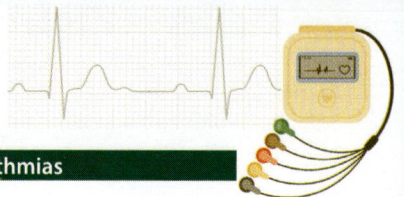

Quadriplet

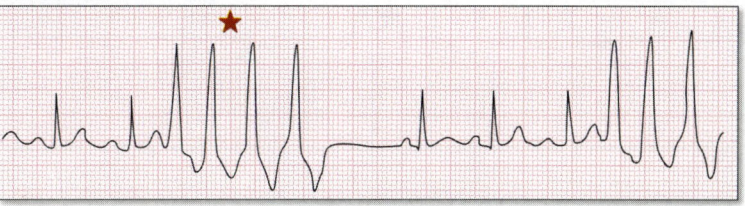

R-on-T phenomenon

- In R-on-T phenomenon, the PVC occurs so early that it falls on the T wave of the preceding beat. Because the cells haven't fully repolarized, ventricular tachycardia or ventricular fibrillation can result (Fig. 9.3).

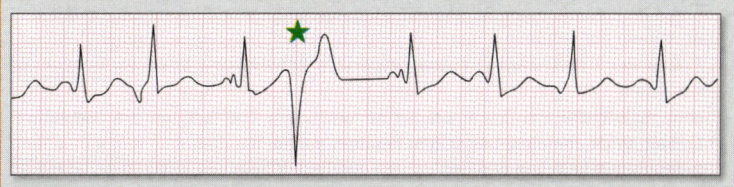

Fig. 9.3 ECG with R on T phenomenon

Uniform PVCs

In uniform PVCs, all PVCs look alike in morphology.

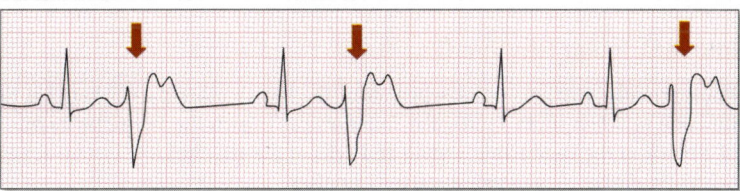

Multiform PVCs

PVCs that look different from one another arise from different sites or from the same site with abnormal conduction. Multiform PVCs may indicate increased ventricular irritability.

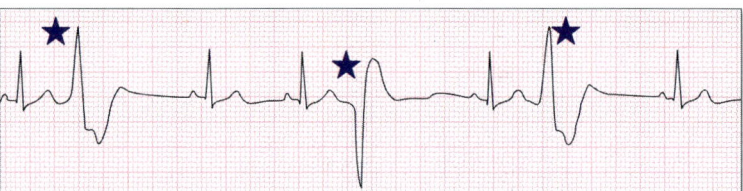

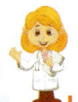

Must Know

- A premature ventricular contraction (PVC) may occur in healthy people without causing problems.
- Not all PVCs require treatment. If there are ≥5 PVCs in one minute, patient needs further intervention.
- PVC can lead to more serious arrhythmias, such as ventricular tachycardia or ventricular fibrillation.
- PVCs also decrease cardiac output, especially if the ectopic beats are frequent or sustained.
- Four main characteristics of premature ventricular contractions: are **Premature**, **Ectopic**, **Wide complexes** and **Compensatory pause**.
- Retrograde P waves may be stimulated by the PVC and cause distortion of the ST segment.
- The PR interval and QT interval aren't measurable on a premature beat. These intervals are measurable only on the normal beats.
- PVCs may be uniform (same form) or multiform (different forms).
- When a PVC strikes on the downslope of the preceding normal T wave—the R-on-T phenomenon—it can trigger more serious rhythm disturbances.

Idioventricular Rhythm (Fig. 9.4)

Idioventricular rhythms occur when all of the heart's other pacemakers fail to function or when supra ventricular impulses can't reach the ventricles because of a block in the conduction system and cells of the His-Purkinje system act as heart's pacemaker to generate electrical impulses.

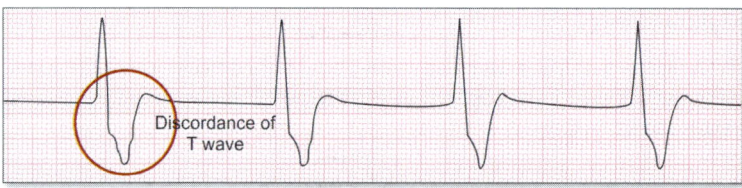

Fig. 9.4 ECG showing idioventricular rhythm

Key Features

- Idioventricular rhythms act as safety mechanisms to prevent ventricular standstill when no impulses are conducted to the ventricles from above the bundle of His.
- These rhythms can occur as ventricular escape beats, idioventricular rhythm, or accelerated idioventricular rhythm.

Characteristics of idioventricular rhythm are given in Table 9.3.

Table 9.3 Characteristics of idioventricular rhythm

ECG Characteristics	**Rhythm**	Atrial rhythm can't be determined. The ventricular rhythm is usually regular
	Atrial rate	Can't be determined.
	Ventricular rate	20 to 40 beats/minute,
	P wave	Absent
	PR interval	Cannot measure
	QRS	Longer than 0.12 second, with a wide and bizarre configuration.
	T wave	Deflection opposite to the direction of QRS complex (Discordance)
	QT interval	Usually prolonged
Causes	The arrhythmias may accompany third-degree heart block or be caused by: • Myocardial ischemia • Myocardial infarction (MI) • Digoxin toxicity • Beta-adrenergic blockers • Pacemaker failure • Metabolic imbalances.	
Signs and Symptoms	Initially may have: • Palpitations • Dizziness, or lightheadedness • Syncopal episode. If the arrhythmia persists, may have: • Hypotension • Weak peripheral pulses • Decreased urine output • Confusion	

Contd...

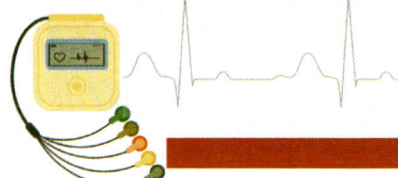

Management	Medical	• Atropine may be prescribed to increase the heart rate. • A pacemaker may be used if atropine isn't effective or if the patient develops hypotension or other signs of instability,
	Nursing	• Patient needs constant assessment and continuous ECG monitoring until treatment restores hemodynamic stability. • If a permanent pacemaker is inserted, teach the patient and his family how it works, how to recognize problems, when to contact the HCWs, and how to monitor pacemaker function.

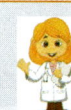

Must Know

Idioventricular rhythms are also called the rhythms of last resort.
• If just one idioventricular beat is generated, it's called a ventricular escape beat.
• Consecutive ventricular beats on the ECG strip make up idioventricular rhythm.
• If the ventricular rate is faster, it's called an accelerated idioventricular rhythm.
• The idioventricular rhythm acts as a safety mechanism to protect the heart from standstill, therefore goal of treatment doesn't include suppressing this rhythm. Idioventricular rhythm should never be treated with lidocaine or other antiarrhythmics that would suppress the safety mechanism as this may lead to cardiac arrest.
• An accelerated idioventricular rhythm has the same characteristics as an idio-ventricular rhythm except that it's faster (rate is 40-100 beats/min) (Fig. 9.5).

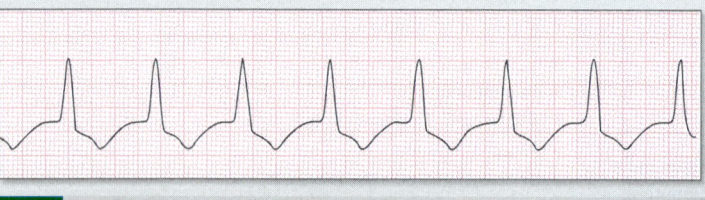

Fig. 9.5 ECG showing accelerated idioventricular rhythm

Ventricular Tachycardia (Figs 9.6A and B)

Ventricular tachycardia (V-tach or VT) is a type of regular and fast heart rate that arises from improper electrical activity in the ventricles of the heart.

Ventricular tachycardia is repetitive firing of an irritable ventricular ectopic focus at a rate of 140 to 250 beats/minutes or more and can lead to cardiac arrest.

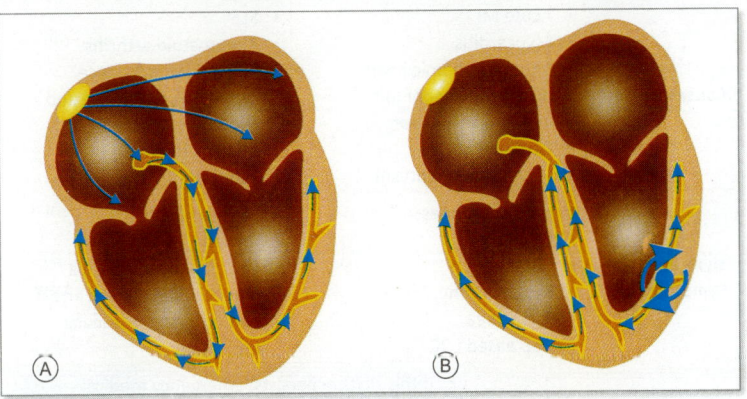

Figs 9.6A and B A. Normal electrical signals; B. Abnormal electrical signals in ventricular arrhythmias

Key Features

- Ventricular tachycardia (V-tach) is a rhythm with a rapid recurrence of premature ventricular contractions with no normal beats in between.
- If this rhythm persists, emergency medical attention is generally required.

Characteristics of ventricular tachycardia have been given in Table 9.4.

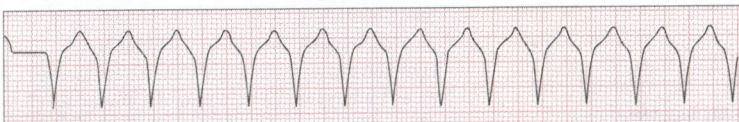

Fig. 9.7 ECG showing ventricular tachycardia

Table 9.4 Characteristics of ventricular tachycardia

ECG Characteristics (Fig. 9.7)	**Rhythm**	Generally regular, on occasions, can be modestly irregular.
	Atrial rate	Cannot be determined
	Ventricular rate	100 to 220 bpm
	P wave	Absent
	PR interval	Cannot be determined
	QRS	Broad and bizarre
	T wave	Cannot be determined
	QT interval	Cannot be determined

Contd...

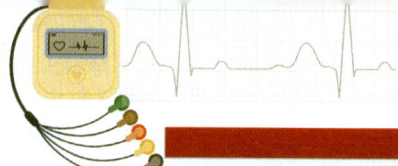

Causes	• Acute MI • Myocarditis • Chronic ischemic heart disease with poor left ventricular function • Cardiomyopathy • Ventricular aneurysm	• SLE • Rheumatoid arthritis • Electrolyte imbalance mainly hypokalaemia and hypomagnaesemia • Digitalis toxicity • Tetralogy of fallot
Signs and Symptoms	• Lightheadedness • Palpitations • Chest pain • Hypotension • Tachypnea • Decreased LOC	• Increased JVP • Anxiety • Ventricular tachycardia may result in cardiac arrest and turn intoventricular fibrillation
Management	**Medical**	• If this rhythm persists, emergency medical attention is generally required. • Defibrillation • Cardioversion • Implantable ICD • Catheter ablation • For those who are stable with a monomorphic waveform the medications procainamide or sotalol may be used and are better than lidocaine • Long-term anti-arrhythmic therapy may be indicated to prevent recurrence of VT. Beta-blockers and a number of class III anti-arrhythmics are commonly used. • As a low magnesium level in the blood is a common cause of VT, magnesium sulfate can be given for torsades de pointes or if a low blood magnesium level is found/suspected.

	Nursing	• Assessing the condition of patient and diagnosis of VT as early as possible.
		• Differentiate between VT with pulse or without pulse.
		• If pulse is present:
		  ■ Provide oxygen
		  ■ Ensure patent IV (preferably x2)
		  ■ Monitor patient very closely
		• If pulseless:
		  ■ Activate Code Blue
		  ■ Begin CPR
		  ■ Defibrillate ASAP
		  ■ Start IV if not already established and hang NS
		  ■ Notify treating doctor
		• Treat reversible causes appropriately (5Ts and 5Hs.)

Comparative features of different types of ventricular tachycardia is depicted below in Table 9.5.

Table 9.5 Comparative features of different types of ventricular tachycardia

Key Features		Monomorphic VT	Polymorphic VT	Torsade de Pointes
Key Features		QRS complexes in monomorphic VT have the same shape and amplitude.	QRS complexes in polymorphic VT vary in shape and amplitude. The QT interval is normal or long.	The QRS reverses polarity and the strip shows a spindle effect. This rhythm is an unusual variant of polymorphic VT with normal or long QT intervals. In French the term means "twisting of the points."
ECG Characteristics	Rhythm	Regular	Regular or irregular	Irregular
	Ventricular rate	100–250 bpm	100–250 bpm	200–250 bpm
	P wave	None or not associated with the QRS	None or not associated with the QRS	None
	PR interval	None	None	None
	QRS	Wide (0.10 sec), bizarre appearance	Wide (0.10 sec), bizarre appearance	Wide (0.10 sec), bizarre appearance

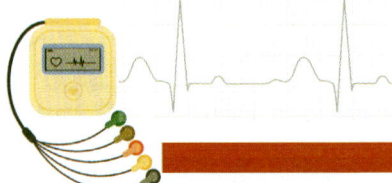

Must Know

- Broad and bizarre QRS complex indicates that QRS complexes are arising from ventricles
- Appearance of normal QRS complex in the middle of ventricular tachycardia
- Fusion beat: This type of complex is caused by two pacemakers, SA node and ventricular pacer. The result is hybrid of fusion complex, which is a complex with some features of both
- Common after MI due to formation of circular course around the ischemic area.
- It is an alarming sign which may progress to ventricular fibrillation and death.
- It is important to confirm the presence or absence of pulses because polymorphic VT may be perfusing or non-perfusing.
- Consider electrolyte abnormalities as a possible etiology.
- In French, Torsades De Pointes means "twisting of the points." It is a distinct type of polymorphic VT. Here the direction of the QRS complex appears to rotate cyclically, pointing downwards for several beats and then twisting and pointing upwards in the same leads.

Ventricular Fibrillation

- Ventricular fibrillation (VF) occurs as a result of multiple weak ectopic foci in the ventricles characterized by no coordinated atrial or ventricular contraction, electrical impulses initiated by multiple ventricular sites and impulses are not transmitted through normal conduction pathway (Figs 9.8A and B).
- Ventricular fibrillation is a chaotic rapid rhythm in which the ventricles quiver and there is no cardiac output.

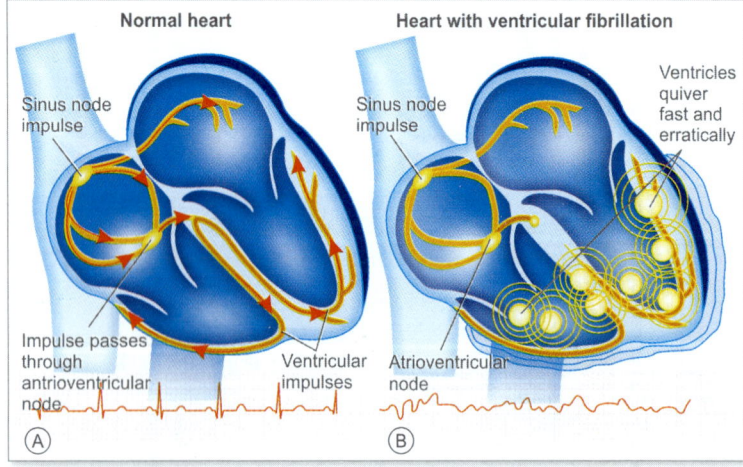

Figs 9.8A and B Ventricular fibrillation: (A) Normal heart beat; (B) Ventricular fibrillation

123

- In VF, Ventricles consist of areas of normal myocardium alternating with areas of ischemic, injured or infarcted myocardium, leading to a chaotic pattern of ventricular depolarization.
- VF is fatal if not successfully terminated within 3 to 5 minutes.

Key Features

- Chaotic electrical activity occurs with no ventricular depolarization or contraction.
- The amplitude and frequency of the fibrillatory activity can be used to define the type of fibrillation as coarse, medium, or fine.
- With V-fib, the ventricles quiver instead of contract, so no pattern or regularity can be detected on the ECG strip.

Characteristics of ventricular fibrillation have been given in Table 9.6.

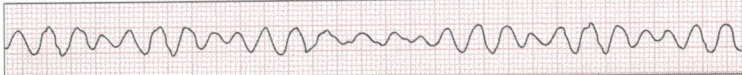

Fig. 9.9 ECG showing ventricular fibrillation

Table 9.6 Characteristics of ventricular fibrillation

ECG Characteristics (Fig. 9.9)	Rhythm	Extremely irregular (Chaotic)
	Atrial rate	Can't be determined
	Ventricular rate	300-600 b/m (Indeterminate)
	P wave	Absent
	PR interval	N/A
	QRS	Fibrillatory baseline
	T wave	Can't be determined.
	QT interval	Can't be determined.
Causes		• Acute coronary syndrome • Stable to unstable VT • PVC'S with R on T phenomenon • Multiple drugs • Electrolyte disturbance • Hypoxia, metabolic acidosis
Signs and Symptoms		• Pulse disappears with onset of VF • Collapse, unconsciousness • Agonal breath/gasping • Onset of reversible death

Contd...

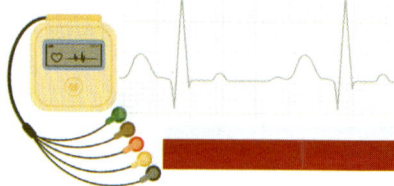

Management	Medical	• Defibrillation • Oxygen, CPR, Intubation • CPR must be performed until the defibrillator arrives to preserve oxygen supply to the brain and other vital organs. • Epinephrine • Amiodarone • Follow algorithm given by AHA
	Nursing	• Activate code blue • Provide CPR to the patient • Administer Medications • Patients and their families need to know when to contact EMS, how to perform CPR, and what long-term therapies are available, such as chronic antiarrhythmic drugs and ICDs

Must Know

Larger, or coarse, fibrillatory waves are easier to convert to a normal rhythm than are smaller waves because larger waves indicate a greater degree of electrical activity in the heart.

Pulseless Electrical Activity

Pulseless Electrical Activity (PEA) encompasses a heterogeneous group of rhythms that are organized or semi organized but lacks a palpable pulse.

Any organized rhythm without a pulse is defined as PEA.

Key Features

• PEA includes idioventricular rhythms, ventricular escape rhythms, post defibrillation idioventricular rhythms. Even sinus rhythm without a detectable pulse is called PEA.
• Pulseless Electrical Activity is considered as a non shockable rhythm.

Characteristics of pulseless electrical activity have been given in Table 9.7.

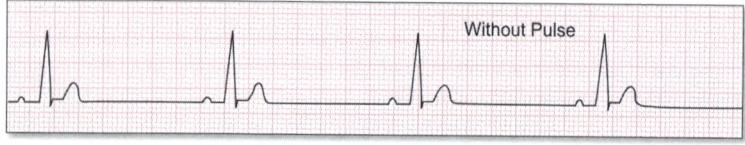

Fig. 9.10 ECG showing pulseless electrical activity

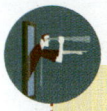

Note

Even an organized electrical activity without a palpable pulse may indicate pulse-less electrical activity.

Table 9.7 Characteristics of pulseless electrical activity

ECG Characteristics (Fig. 9.10)	Rhythm	Depends on whether PEA is associated with idioventricular rhythms, ventricular escape rhythms, post defibrillation idioventricular rhythms or even sinus rhythm.	
	Atrial rate		
	Ventricular rate		
	P wave		
	PR interval		
	QRS		
	T wave		
	QT interval		
Causes	• Hypovolemia		• Hypoxia
Signs and Symptoms	• No pulse • Unresponsiveness • Organized rhythm on the monitor		
Management	Medical	• Start CPR • Give epinephrine1mg IV/IO (repeat every 3-5 minutes) • Consider advanced airway and capnography	

	Nursing	• Recognize this life-threatening arrhythmia and start resuscitation right away
		• Remember that shock is not given in this condition.
		• Follow algorithm given by AHA or Indian guidelines:
		  ■ If a palpable pulse is present and rhythm is organized (during rhythm check), begin post cardiac arrest care.
		  ■ Identify and correct an underlying cause if present.	

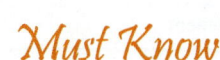

Must Know

• Previously, electromechanical dissociation (EMD) term was used to describe patients who displayed electrical activity on the cardiac monitor but lacked apparent contractile function because of an undetectable pulse.
• VF, pVT and asystole are pulseless rhythms excluded by definition of PEA.
• Pulseless electrical activity can lead to asystole.

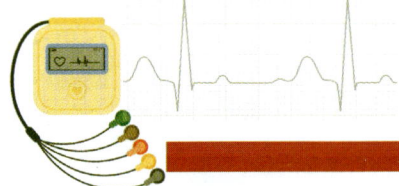

Agonal Rhythm

Agonal rhythm is when the idioventricular rhythm is 20 beats or less per minute.

Key Features

Agonal rhythm is frequently seen as the last-ordered semblance of a heart rhythm when resuscitation efforts are unsuccessful.

Characteristics of agonal rhythm have been given in Table 9.8.

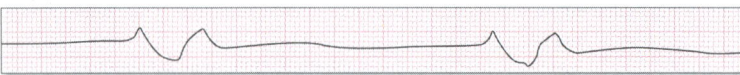

Fig. 9.11 ECG showing agonal rhythm

Table 9.8 Characteristics of agonal rhythm

ECG Characteristics (Fig. 9.11)	**Rhythm**	Usually regular
	Atrial rate	Cannot be seen
	Ventricular rate	Very slow, <20 bpm
	P wave	Absent
	PR interval	Not measurable
	QRS	Wide and bizarre (>0.12 sec)
	T wave	T wave deflection
Causes	• Trauma • Acute MI • Natural progression to death	
Signs and Symptoms	• Loss of consciousness • No palpable pulse or measurable BP	
Management	**Medical**	• Follow CPR/ACLS Protocol • If lifesaving efforts have already been attempted no further treatment

	Nursing	• Make sure there aren't any loose leads or leads that have come off the patient
		• Call a Code Blue
		• Start CPR
		• Notify the treating doctor
		• If death is the expected outcome:
		  ▪ Monitor vital signs
		  ▪ Record rhythm progression
		  ▪ Support family and friends

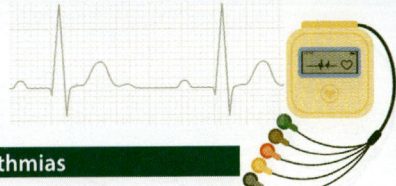

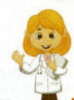

Must Know

- An agonal heart rhythm is a variant of asystole.
- The QRS complex of an agonal rhythm is usually very wide and could be wider than an idioventricular rhythm.
- Agonal heart rhythm is usually ventricular in origin. Occasional P waves and QRS complexes can be seen on the electrocardiogram.

Asystole

Asystole is a dire form of cardiac arrest in which the heart stops beating and there is no electrical activity in the heart. As a result, the heart is at a total standstill.

Key Features

- Characterized by total absence of ventricular electrical activity.
- Asystole has been called the arrhythmia of death. The patient is in cardiopulmonary arrest. Without rapid initiation of CPR and appropriate treatment, the situation quickly becomes irreversible.

Characteristics of asystole have been given in Table 9.9.

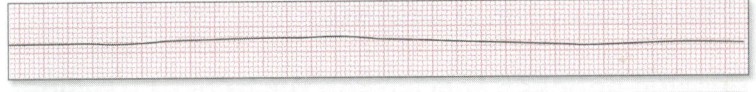

Fig. 9.12 ECG showing asystole

Table 9.9 Characteristics of asystole

	Rhythm	
	Atrial rate	
	Ventricular rate	
ECG Characteristics (Fig. 9.12)	P wave	Asystole looks like a nearly **flat line** on the ECG strip except for changes caused by chest compressions during CPR.
	PR interval	
	QRS	
	T wave	
	QT interval	
Causes	• Drug intoxication such as cocaine overdose • Cardiac tamponade • Hypothermia prolonged hypoxemia • Severe, uncorrected acid-base disturbances	• Electric shock • MI • Severe electrolyte disturbances such as hyperkalemia • Massive pulmonary embolism

Contd...

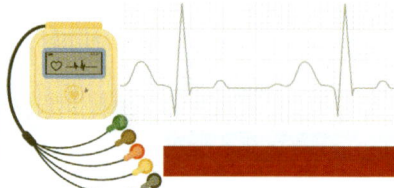

Signs and Symptoms		• Diminished pulse or blood pressure • Unresponsiveness
Management	Medical	• Start CPR • Give epinephrine 1 mg IV/IO (repeat every 3-5 minutes) • Endotracheal intubation • Transcutaneous pacing • Identify and either treat or remove the underlying cause.
	Nursing	• Recognize this life-threatening arrhythmia and start resuscitation right away • Follow algorithm given by AHA or Indian guidelines. • Treatment of reversible causes of asystole.

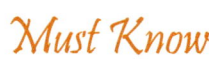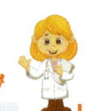

Must Know

- A patient with pacemaker may also have asystole in whom pacer spikes may be evident on the ECG strip, but no P wave or QRS complex occurs in response to the stimulus.
- Pulse less electrical activity can lead to asystole.

NURSING PROCESS APPLIED FOR THE PATIENT HAVING VENTRICULAR ARRHYTHMIAS

Decreased Cardiac Output

Nursing Assessment

Decreased level of consciousness, cool peripheries, increased JVP, hypoxemia, palpitations, hypotension or syncope, tachypnea, agonal breath/ gasping, unconsciousness, unresponsiveness.

Nursing Diagnosis

Decreased cardiac, cerebral, and peripheral tissue perfusion related to altered electrical conduction as evidenced by dizziness, decreased level of consciousness, chest pain, shortness of breath, pulselessness, apnea, shock, and/or cardiopulmonary arrest

Planning

- To achieve adequate cardiac output, cerebral and peripheral tissue perfusion.
- To eradicate or decrease the incidence of the ventricular dysrhythmia

Nursing Interventions

- Monitor vital signs, palpate pulses, note significant variations in the Blood Pressure.
- Check changes in skin color, temperature.
- Assess level of consciousness and sensorium.
- Monitor urine output.
- Auscultate heart sounds, noting rate, rhythm, presence of extra heartbeats, dropped beats.
- Assess SpO_2 using pulse oximetry.
- Obtain 12 lead ECG and interpret the rhythm.
- If the patient is not in full arrest, maintain Airway, Breathing and Circulation. Low-flow oxygen by nasal cannula or mask may decrease the rate of PVCs. Higher flow rates are usually needed for the patient with VT, and if pulseless VT or VF occurs, the patient needs immediate endotracheal intubation, and support of breathing with a manual resuscitator bag.
- If the patient is in full arrest, use current cardiopulmonary resuscitation guidelines. As in case of ventricular fibrillation or pulseless ventricular tachycardia.
- The most important intervention for a patient with pulseless VT or VF is rapid defibrillation. If a defibrillator is not available, and the arrest was witnessed, begin chest compressions and, as soon as possible defibrillate the patient. Maintain CPR between all other interventions (other than rhythm check and shock delivery) for patients without adequate breathing and circulation.
- Insert and maintain IV access.
- Administer epinephrine, amiodarone or other antiarrhythmic medication depending on type of arrhythmia as prescribed by the physician.
- If the patient has electrolyte imbalances, or they are suspected, supplemental potassium, calcium, and/or magnesium is administered IV as prescribed.Long-term management may be done by Implantable Cardioverter Defibrillator (ICDs).
- Manage the patient with asystole or PEA with CPR. Initiate CPR, prepare for intubation, provide oxygenated breathing with a manual resuscitator bag, and administer epinephrine every 3 to 5 minutes in an attempt to have the patient regain an effective cardiac rhythm.
- Reassess the pulse and rhythm to check the effectiveness of interventions performed

Evaluation

Expected patient outcomes may include:
- Maintains cardiac output
- Demonstrates heart rate, blood pressure, respiratory rate and level of consciousness within normal ranges
- Demonstrates no or decreased episodes of dysrhythmia

Anxiety

Nursing Assessment

Palpitations, tachypnea, restlessness, anxiety.

Nursing Diagnosis

Anxiety related to fear of the unknown.

Planning

To minimize the anxiety of patient

Nursing Interventions

- Remain with the patient to ensure rest and to allay anxiety
- Provide quiet and calm environment.
- For some patients with asymptomatic short runs of PVCs, strategies to reduce stress help limit the incidence of the dysrhythmia.
- Make a trustworthy therapeutic relation with the patient. Encourage patient to ventilate his feelings regarding disease condition and provide counseling to the patient.
- Promote a sense of confidence in patient to live with a dysrhythmia. The nursing goal is to maximize the patient's control and to make the unknown less threatening.

Evaluation

Expected patient outcomes may include:
- Experiences reduced anxiety
- Expresses a positive attitude about living with the dysrhythmia
- Expresses confidence in one'e own abilities to take appropriate actions in an emergency.

Deficient Knowledge

Nursing Assessment

Frequent questioning by patient and his/her family members

Nursing Diagnosis

Deficient knowledge about ventricular dysrhythmias and its treatment as evidenced by frequent questioning by patient and his/her family members.

Planning

To provide knowledge about the dysrhythmia and its treatment

Nursing Interventions

- Patients who experience dysrhythmias are often facing alterations in their lifestyle and job functions. Provide information about the dysrhythmia, the precipitating factors, and mechanisms to limit the dysrhythmia.
- If the patient is placed on medications, teach the patient and significant others the dosage, route, action, and side effects. Explain to the patient the importance of taking all medications.
- If the patient needs periodic laboratory work to monitor the effects of the medications (e.g., serum electrolytes or drug levels), discuss with the patient the frequency of these laboratory visits and where to have the tests drawn. Discuss methods for the patient to remember to take the medications, such as numbered medication boxes or linking the medications with other activities such as meals or sleep.
- Make sure the patient understands the schedule for the next physician's checkup.
- If the patient is at risk for electrolyte imbalance, teach the patient any dietary considerations to prevent electrolyte depletion of vital substances.
- Teach the patient to reduce the amount of caffeine intake in the diet.
- Explain the need to read the ingredients of over-the-counter medications to limit caffeine intake.
- If appropriate, encourage the patient to become involved in an exercise program or a smoking-cessation group.
- Stress the importance of stress reduction and smoking cessation. If the patient has a pacemaker or an ICD, provide teaching about the settings, signs of pacemaker failure (dizziness, syncope, palpitations, fast or slow pulse rate), and when to notify the physician.
- Explain any environmental hazards based on the manufacturer's recommendations, such as heavy machinery and airport security checkpoints.
- Make sure the patient understands the schedule for the next physician's checkup.
- If the patient has an ICD, encourage the patient to keep a diary of the number of times the device discharges.
- Teach the patient how to take the pulse and recognize an irregular rhythm.
- Explain that the patient needs to notify the healthcare provider when symptoms such as irregular pulse, chest pain, shortness of breath, and dizziness occur.
- CPR training may be given to family members of patient.

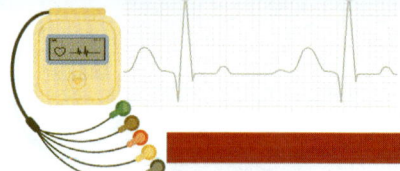

Evaluation

Expected patient outcomes may include:

- Expresses understanding of the dysrhythmia and its treatment
- Explains the dysrhythmia and its effects Describes the medication regimen and its rationale
- Explains the need for therapeutic serum level of the medication
- Describes a plan to eradicate or limit factors that contribute to the occurrence of the dysrhythmia
- States actions to take in the event of an emergency

Practice Questions

1. **Which ECG finding is most likely to be seen at the time of cardiac arrest?**

   a. Atrial flutter   b. Atrial fibrillation

   c. Ventricular tachycardia   d. Ventricular fibrillation

2. **Identify the rhythm**

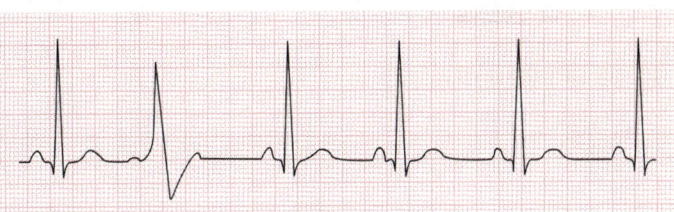

3. **Identify the rhythm**

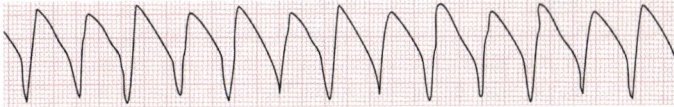

4. **Identify the rhythm**

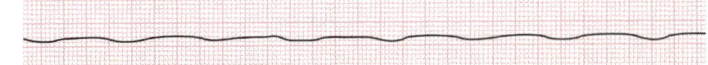

5. **All of the following are features of premature ventricular complex except:**

   a. Wide QRS complex

   b. Absent P wave

   c. Complete compensatory pause

   d. Prolonged PR interval

6. **Identify the rhythm**

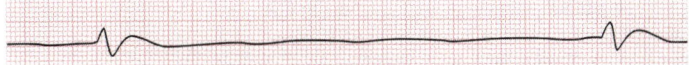

7. **A 60-year-old patient clutches chest and falls down. A nurse arrives on the scene. What is the first thing to be done by the nurse.**

   a. Check peripheral pulse   b. Chest compressions

   c. Clear patient airway   d. Call for help

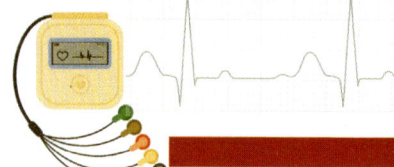
8. Identify the rhythm

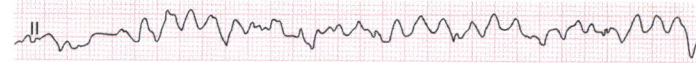

9. Identify the rhythm

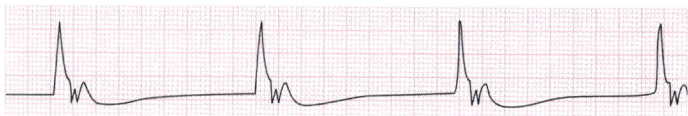

10. Identify the rhythm

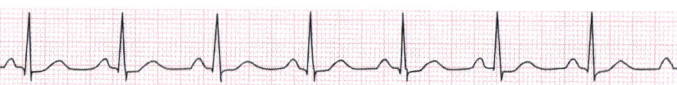

11. What is the correct sequence of events according to BLS.
a. Start CPR, give rescue breaths, assess pulse
b. Give rescue breaths, check pulse, start CPR
c. Assess patient, activate emergency response system, call for defibrillator and start CPR
d. Assess pulse, defibrillate, start CPR

12. In ventricular tachycardia, extra systoles appears in:
a. P wave   b. QRS complex
c. T wave   d. R wave

13. An unresponsive patient is brought to the emergency department with no proper history. What will be your next step?
a. Check for carotid pulse
b. Check for responsiveness
c. Secure airway
d. Provide shock of 300 joules

14. If a PVC falls on _____wave, it could lead to serious arrhythmias. This is known as _____on _____ phenomenon.
a. T; RT   b. R; TU
c. T; ST   d. P; QR

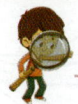

Answers

1. d
2. Premature ventricular contraction
3. Ventricular Tachycardia
4. Asystole
5. d
6. Agonal Rhythm
7. d
8. Ventricular Fibrillation
9. Idioventricular rhythm
10. Pulseless Electrical Activity
11. c
12. b
13. a
14. a

Heart Blocks

Chapter 10

INTRODUCTION

Heart block is a type of bradycardia (too-slow heartbeat) that is also called atrioventricular, or **AV block.** In this condition, the electrical signals that stimulate heart muscle contractions are partially or totally blocked between the upper chambers (atria) and the lower chambers (ventricles).

KEY FEATURES

- Relationship between the P waves and QRS complexes determines the atrioventricular (AV) conduction.
- Normally, there is a P wave that precedes each QRS complex by a fixed PR interval of 0.12 to 0.20 seconds.
- Physiologically, this time interval of 0.12 to 0.20 second allows the atria to pump blood into the ventricles, before ventricles contract, by delaying conduction to AV node.
- When there is a delay or disturbance, i.e. >0.20 seconds in the transmission of an impulse from the atria to the ventricles, it is called AV Block.
- Causes may be attributed to **anatomical or functional impairment** in the heart's conduction system.
- This disruption in normal electrical activity can be transient or permanent, and then further characterized as delayed, intermittent, or absent.
- In general, there are three degrees of AV nodal blocks: first degree, second degree (Mobitz type 1 or 2), and third degree.

FIRST DEGREE ATRIOVENTRICULAR BLOCK

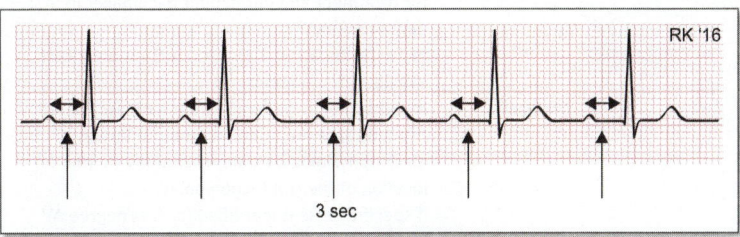

3 sec

Fig. 10.1 ECG showing first degree atrioventricular block

Characteristics of first degree atrioventricular block have been given in Table 10.1.

Table 10.1 Characteristics of first degree atrioventricular block

ECG Characteristics (Fig. 10.1)	Rhythm	Regular
	Atrial rate	60 – 100 beats/min, depends on underlying rhythm
	Ventricular rate	60 – 100 beats/min depends on underlying rhythm
	P wave	Normal
	PR interval	Greater than >0.20 seconds without disruption of atrial to ventricular conduction PR interval measurement is constant.
	QRS	Normal
	P:QRS	1:1
	T wave	Normal
	QT interval	Normal
Causes		• Fibrotic changes of the cardiac conduction • Increased vagal tone (in younger patients)system (elderly patients) • Coronary Heart Disease • Myocardial Infarction • Inflammation • Infiltrative Diseases • And Neuromuscular Disorders
Signs and Symptoms		• Generally asymptomatic and without significant complications. • Till PR interval is shorter than 0.30 seconds, prolonged conduction is well tolerated • As PR interval increases beyond 0.30 seconds, synchronization of atria and ventricles contraction worsens and may results in dizziness, fatigue and dyspnea. • First degree AV block is not actually a block but a delay in impulse conduction.

Contd...

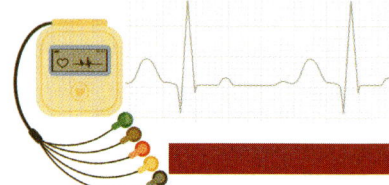

Management	Medical	• For majority patients there is no recommendation for treatment and permanent pacemaker in first degree AV blocks. • In asymptomatic patients, no further diagnostic evaluation is required. • In symptomatic patients, those with associated heart disease are referred for more invasive electrophysiologic studies to identifying the location of the conduction delay. • If specific cause is identified for first degree AV block, treatment focuses on eliminating it
	Nursing	• It focuses on identification of patients at risk of developing atrioventricular bocks by taking complete medical history especially elderly patients. • First-degree AV blocks are less likely to cause hemodynamic instability and usually require only monitoring for progression. • First degree AV blocks with normal QRS complexes usually have good prognosis if identified. Those with wide QRS may indicate need to monitor and may progress to advanced type block. Therefore, look for changes in QRS morphology while monitoring ECG.

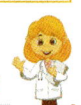

Must Know

- First degree AV block may progress to further second degree AV block or complete heart block.
- In first degree AV block rate is not altered by the presence of the prolonged PR interval because it is still being controlled by the SA node.

SECOND DEGREE ATRIOVENTRICULAR BLOCK (AV) (FIG. 10.2)

- Second degree AV block is diagnosed when one or more atrial impulses from SA node fails to conduct or pass through AV node to the ventricles.
- Some of the atrial impulses are blocked completely.
- The PR interval progresses until there is no conduction or a skipped beat appears and the process is repeated.
- It is broadly of two types – Mobitz's type I (Fig. 10.3) or Wencheback's; Mobitz's type II.
- The other types are P:QRS ratios, 2:1 AV block

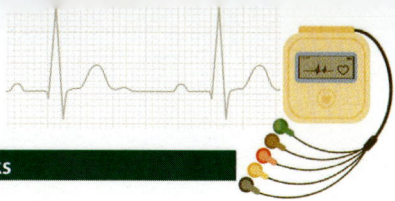

Second Degree AV Block – Mobitz's Type I (Fig. 10.2)

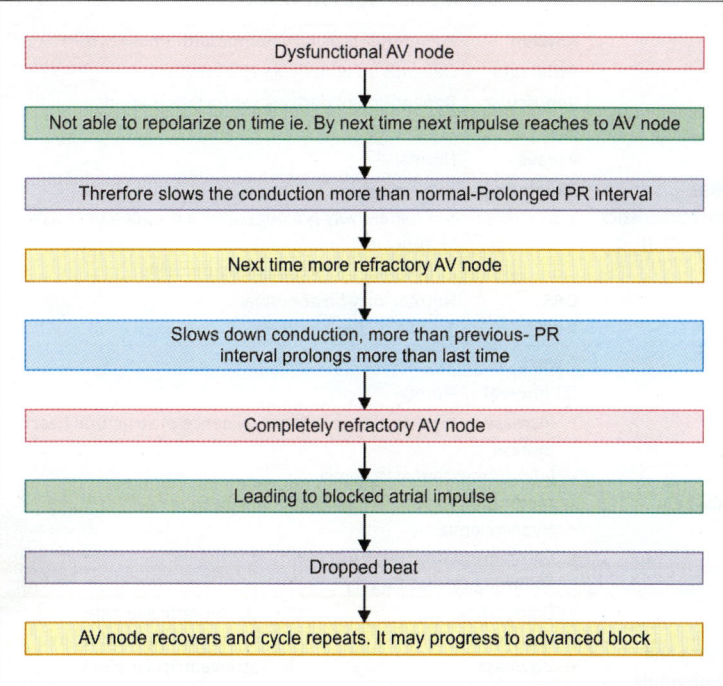

Fig. 10.2 Pathogenesis of 2nd degree AV block – Mobitz's Type I (Wenckebach)

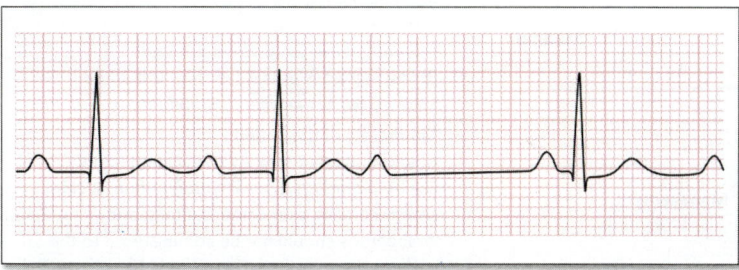

Fig. 10.3 ECG showing Mobitz Type I AV block

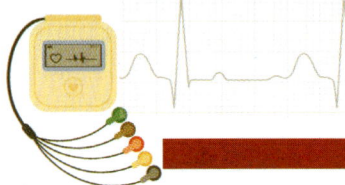

The characteristics of Mobitz Type I AV block have been given in Table 10.2

Table 10.2 Characteristics of Mobitz Type I AV block

ECG Characteristics (Fig. 10.3)	**Rhythm**	P-P interval is usually normal with sinus rhythm
	Atrial rate	Depends on underlying atrial rhythm
	Ventricular rate	Depends on underlying ventricular rhythm
	P wave	Normal
	PR interval	• >0.20sec • Progressively prolongs, until a dropped beat (QRS) appears. • Irregular PR Interval measurements
	QRS	Normal, may be abnormal
	P:QRS	3:2, 4:3, 5:4 and so forth
	T wave	Normal
	QT interval	Normal
Causes	• Increase or high vagal tone without evidence of structural heart disease • Inferior myocardial ischemia • Medication toxicity (AV nodal blocking agents) • Hyperkalemia • Cardiomyopathy (Lyme disease) • Following cardiac surgery	
Signs and Symptoms	• Bradycardia • Hypotension • Dizziness • Confusion • Syncope	• Diaphoretic and pale • Chest pain (second-degree atrioventricular block secondary to myocardial ischemia).
Management	**Medical**	• Treatment for a Mobitz type I (Wenckebach) is often not necessary • Atropine • If unresponsive to atropine, pacing (transcutaneous or transvenous) should be initiated for hemodynamic stabilization
	Nursing	• Monitoring of the patient • Medications that slow AV nodal conduction like beta-blockers, non-dihydropyridine calcium channel blocks, adenosine, digitalis, and amiodarone should not be administered to the patients, if prescribed, then should be discussed with the physician • Do not do any nursing intervention that may cause vagal nerve stimulation like gag reflex, or administration of enemas etc. Vagal stimulation may decrease the HR further progressing to advanced block. Same is applicable in all types of blocks.

Contd...

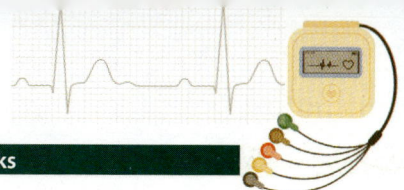

141

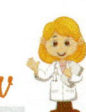

Must Know

- Mobitz type 1 is often a benign rhythm.
- Most patients are asymptomatic, and there is tendency of minimal hemodynamic disturbance.

Second Degree AV Block – Mobitz's Type II (Table 10.3)

In second-degree Mobitz type 2 AV block, there are intermittent non-conducted P waves without warning.

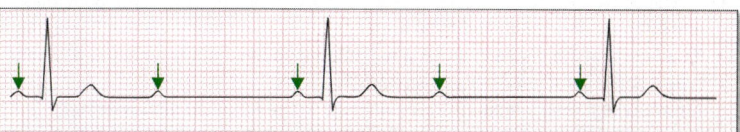

Fig. 10.4 ECG showing Mobitz Type II AV block

The characteristics of Mobitz Type II AV block have been given in Table 10.3.

Table 10.3 Characteristics of Mobitz Type II AV block

ECG Characteristics (Fig. 10.4)	**Rhythm**	P-P interval is usually normal with sinus rhythm
	Atrial rate	Depends on underlying atrial rhythm
	Ventricular rate	Depends on underlying ventricular rhythm and P:QRS ratio
	P wave	Normal
	PR interval	PR interval is constant for those P waves just before QRS complexes
	QRS	Usually abnormal but may be normal also
	P:QRS	2:1, 3:1, 4:1, 5:1, and so forth
	T wave	Normal
	QT interval	Normal
Causes		• Mobitz type II is rarely seen in patients without structural heart disease • Often associated with myocardial ischemia and fibrosis or sclerosis of the myocardium.
Signs and Symptoms		• Syncope • Dizziness • Chest pain • Hypotension • Diaphoretic

Contd...

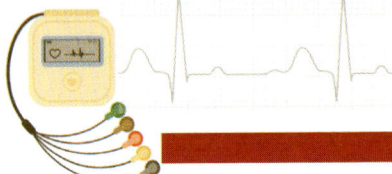
| Management | Medical | • Initiating pacing as soon as this rhythm is identified.
• Transvenous pacing
• Permanent pacemaker
• Often do not respond to atropine |
| | Nursing | • As soon as the patient is diagnosed with this conduction block, prepare the articles for trans venous pacing as prescribed by physician |

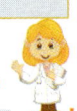

Must Know

- In Mobitz type II, there is a constant PR interval across the rhythm strip both before and after the non-conducted atrial beat.
- Be aware that if more than one P wave is not conducted this is no longer a Mobitz type II and is considered a high degree AV block.
- Mobitz type II blocks imply structural damage to the AV conduction system.
- This rhythm often progresses to third-degree atrioventricular block.
- **High-grade AV block** is a form of second-degree (incomplete) heart block that can commonly be confused with third-degree (complete) heart block. It occurs when there are two or more consecutively blocked P waves. The P:QRS is 3:1 or higher and the ventricular rate is typically very slow.
- **High-grade AV block** is differentiated from the third-degree (complete) heart block by there remains some relationship between the P waves and QRS complexes. In other words, there is still some AV conduction taking place.
- **2:1 AV block** - When a Mobitz type I has a fixed conduction ratio of 2:1 i.e. 2 conducted beats to one non-conducted beat, it is difficult to differentiate between type I and type II. Referred as 2:1 AV block. This should be managed like a type II with transcutaneous or transvenous pacing.

THIRD DEGREE AV BLOCK – COMPLETE HEART BLOCK

In third degree AV block or complete heart block there is absence of AV nodal conduction i.e. no atrial impulses are conducted through the AV node (Fig. 10.5).

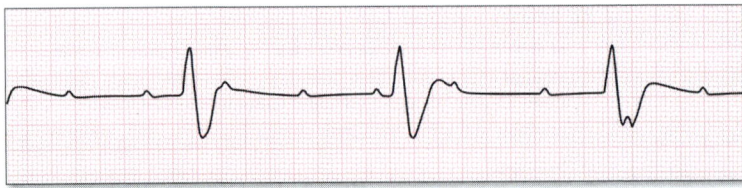

Fig. 10.5 ECG showing 3rd degree AV Block

Characteristics of 3rd degree AV block have been given in Table 10.4.

Table 10.4 Characteristics of 3rd degree AV Block

ECG Characteristics (Fig. 10.5)	**Rhythm**	The PP interval is regular and the RR interval is regular; but the PP interval is not equal to the RR interval.
	Atrial rate	Depends on the escape and underlying atrial rhythm
	Ventricular rate	Depends on the escape and underlying ventricular rhythm Usually between 20 – 40 bpm
	P wave	Depends on underlying rhythm
	PR interval	Very irregular
	QRS	Depends on the escape rhythm; in junctional escape, QRS shape and duration are usually normal, and in ventricular escape, QRS shape and duration are usually abnormal.
Causes		• Same causes as of Mobitz type I and type II • Inferior MI, degeneration of the conduction system • AV-nodal blocking agents such as beta-blockers, non-dihydropyridine calcium channel blockers, adenosine, digitalis and amiodarone.
Signs and Symptoms		• Syncope • Hypotension • Dizziness • Diaphoretic • Chest pain
Management	**Medical**	• Urgent hospital admission for cardiac monitoring • Backup temporary cardiac pacing (transvenous pacing), and insertion of a permanent pacemaker.
	Nursing	• Monitor patient's vitals and continuous cardiac monitoring to be done and documented • As soon as the patient is diagnosed with this conduction block, prepare the articles for trans venous pacing or permanent pacing as prescribed by physician • Educate patient and family about permanent pacemaker care.

Must Know

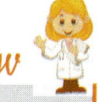

• AV dissociation occurs when there is no relationship between the P waves and QRS complexes.
• Patients with complete heart block are at great risk of developing asystole, ventricular tachycardia, and sudden cardiac death. Insertion of a permanent pacemaker is required.

INTERVENTRICULAR CONDUCTION DELAYS/DEFECTS [BUNDLE BRANCH BLOCKS (BBB) AND FASCICULAR BLOCKS/HEMI BLOCKS]

The BBB and hemiblocks comes under the interventricular conduction delay or defect.

The interventricular conduction comprises primarily of bundle of His, bundle branches –left and right, anterior and posterior fascicles of left bundle branch and purkinje fibers. Impulse through the bundle of His, bundle branches, through fascicles reaches the purkinje fibers which is in the sub endocardium, transmits the impulse to the cardiomyocytes, thereby allowing all the cardiomyocytes to contract simultaneously. The interventricular septum receives Purkinje fibres from the left bundle.

Whenever there is any block in the interventricular conduction, it leads to bundle branch blocks or fascicular blocks.

When there is a bundle branch-**LBBB (left bundle branch blocks) or RBBB (right bundle branch blocks)**, electrical activation of ventricle is awaited, till it is activated by the opposite ventricle.

The block in the interventricular conduction, appears as change in QRS complex morphology.

Normal Mechanism of Interventricular Conduction (Fig. 10.6)

- Normally ventricular depolarization initiates from interventricular septum, which receives purkinje fibres from left bundle branch.

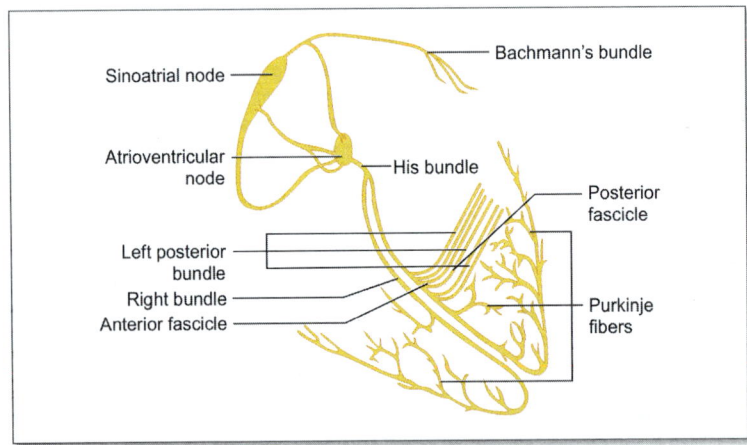

Fig. 10.6 Interventricular conduction

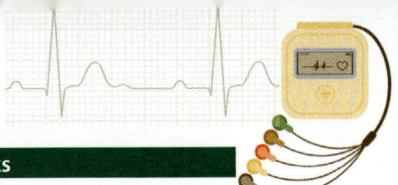

- Depolarization of left part of interventricular septum occurs first then moving to right side.
- Normally septum depolarizes from left to right nut in LBBB reverse happens i.e. right to left septum depolarization
- The septum depolarization generates small r wave in V1-V2 and small q waves in V5-V6, also called as septal q waves (Fig. 10.7).

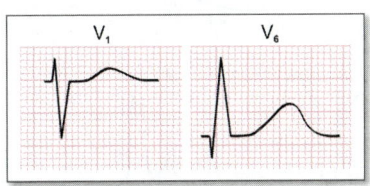

Fig. 10.7 Small r wave in V1 and q wave in V6

Bundle branch block may be complete (i.e. QRS >0.12 sec) or incomplete (QRS duration <0.12 sec).

Left Bundle Branch Block (LBBB) (Table 10.5)

- LBBB is one of the most common electro physiological abnormality. LBBB is mostly pathologic, associated with cardiac diseases – myocardial ischemia, hypertrophy, etc.
- When ventricular hypertrophy occurs it causes stretching and separation of Purkinje fibres thereby causing delay and ineffective ventricular depolarization.

LBBB Mechanism

- Due to block in left bundle branch, the septum depolarizes from right to left, leading to disappearance of normal r wave in V1-V2 and q waves in V5-V6 (Fig. 10.8).
- Thus there is delayed and slow stimulation of left ventricle and ventricular stimulation is directed towards left chest leads (Fig. 10.8).
- Characteristic wide S wave in V1-V2 (QS complex), may be notched appearing as **W** and broad, clumsy R wave, may be notched in V5-V6, appearing as **M.** (Fig. 10.8).

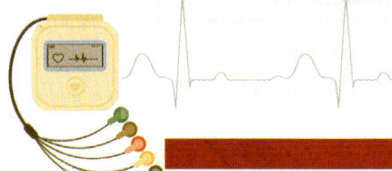

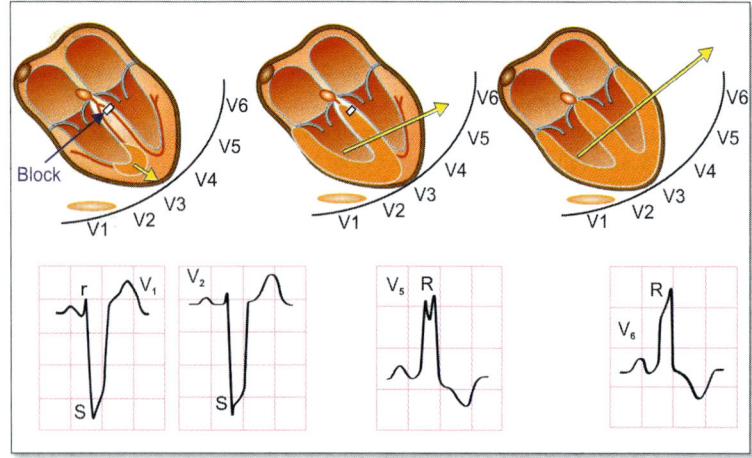

Fig. 10.8 Conduction in LBBB and its characteristics waves

The characteristics of LBBB have been given in Table 10.5.

Table 10.5 Characteristics of left bundle branch block

ECG Characteristics	Rhythm	Regular
	Atrial rate	Depends on underlying atrial rhythm
	Ventricular rate	Depends on underlying ventricular rhythm
	P wave	Normal
	PR interval	Regular
	QT interval	In complete LBBB QRS = >0.12 second Incomplete LBBB QRS = 0.10–0.12 second
	QRS	>0.12 sec
	Lead V1	Either a QS or a small r wave with deep broad S wave, which may be broad and resemble "W"
	Lead V6	Notched R wave and no Q wave, often resembles "M"

Contd...

Causes	• Myocardial ischemia • Hypertrophy of myocardium • Dilated cardiomyopathy • Heart failure • Infective causes	• Infiltrative diseases like amyloidosis • Hypertension • Myocarditis • Valvular heart diseases
Signs and Symptoms	• Usually asymptomatic • No sign and symptoms • Only identified in ECG	
Management	**Medical**	• No specific treatment • Treatment of underlying disorder needs to be done • In heart failure patients CRT i.e. cardiac re synchronization therapy to pace both the ventricles together, to prevent any complications in Heart failure patients.
	Nursing	• Monitor patient's vitals and continuous cardiac monitoring to be done and documented.

Must Know

- There will be often accompanying ST segment changes with LBBB, because when depolarization of ventricles is abnormal, there will be abnormality in repolarization also.
- LBBB is mostly pathologic; you will find an associated cardiac disease with it. Therefore, always take a good history to correlate ECG findings.
- CRT does not treat LBBB, it only helps to pace ventricles together thereby reducing adverse life threatening cardiac events in HF patients.
- LBBB affects the early phases of ventricular activation, whereas RBBB affects the terminal phase of ventricular activation
- Remember pneumonic **WILLIAM** – W pattern in V1-V2 and M pattern in V5-V6 in LBBB

Right Bundle Branch Block (RBBB) (Table 10.6)

- In RBBB, the right ventricle is activated after the left ventricle.
- RBBB is not associated with cardiovascular risk factors like LBBB, but may be associated with structural changes from myocardial stretch or ischemia.

RBBB Mechanism

- When the right bundle branch is blocked, electrical stimuli from the atrioventricular (AV) conducts (goes through) and down to the left bundle branch.
- The left ventricle depolarizes first while the right ventricle polarizes later, causing the characteristic ECG findings (Fig. 10.9).
  - QRS duration is greater than or equal to 120 milliseconds
  - RSR` pattern in leads V1 and V2
  - S wave is of greater duration than the R in V6

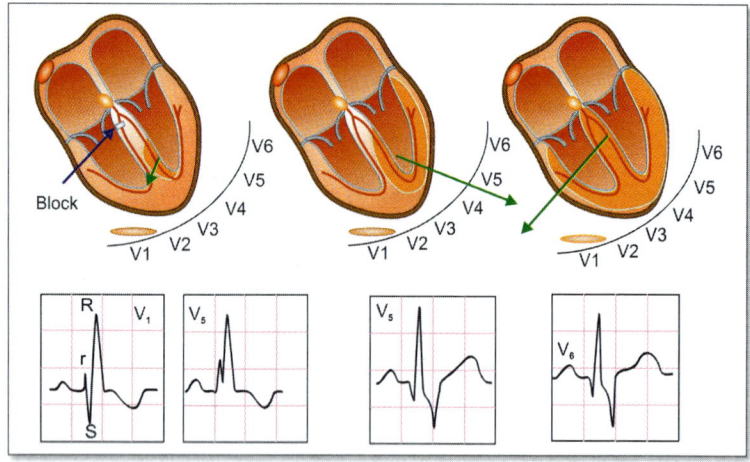

The characteristics of RBBB have been given in Table 10.6.

Table 10.6 Characteristics of right bundle branch block

ECG Characteristics (Fig. 10.9)	Rhythm	Regular	
	Atrial rate	Depends on underlying atrial rhythm	
	Ventricular rate	Depends on underlying ventricular rhythm	
	P wave	Normal	
	PR interval	Regular	
	QT interval	In complete RBBB QRS = >0.12 second Incomplete RBBB QRS = 0.10–0.12 second	
	QRS	>0.12 sec	
	Lead V1	rSR' pattern in V1	V1 rSR'
	Lead V6	qRs in V6	V6 qRs

Contd...

Causes	• Idiopathic- scarring or fibrosis of right bundle • Congenital heart diseases • Acute cor pulmonale • Cardiac surgery • COPD • Right Ventricular hypertrophy • Iatrogenic (right heart catheterization)	
Signs and Symptoms	• Usually asymptomatic • No sign and symptoms • Only identified in ECG	
Management	Medical	• No specific treatment • Treatment of underlying disorder needs to be done if associated with any cardiac disease
	Nursing	• Monitor patient's vitals and documentation.

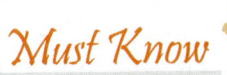

Must Know

• Asymptomatic and isolated RBBB usually don't require any evaluation
• Remember pneumonic **MARROW** – M pattern in V1-V2 and W pattern in V6 in RBBB

Fascicular Blocks

• Fascicular blocks also referred as hemiblocks are associated with interruption in left and right fascicles that originates from the left bundle branch.
• Blockage in anterior fascicle causes left anterior fascicle block (LAFB)
• Blockage in posterior fascicle causes left posterior fascicle block (LPFB)
• The **QRS duration** in fascicular blocks prolongs but does not extend 0.12 sec.
• In fascicular block there is electrical axis deviation:
  ▪ LAFB = left axis deviation = –45° to – 90°
  ▪ LPFB = right axis deviation = +90° to +180°
• Bifascicular block is when LAFB or LPFB is accompanied with RBBB
• LPFB features rs complexes in leads i and avl and qr complexes in II, III, and aVF. (Fig. 10.10)

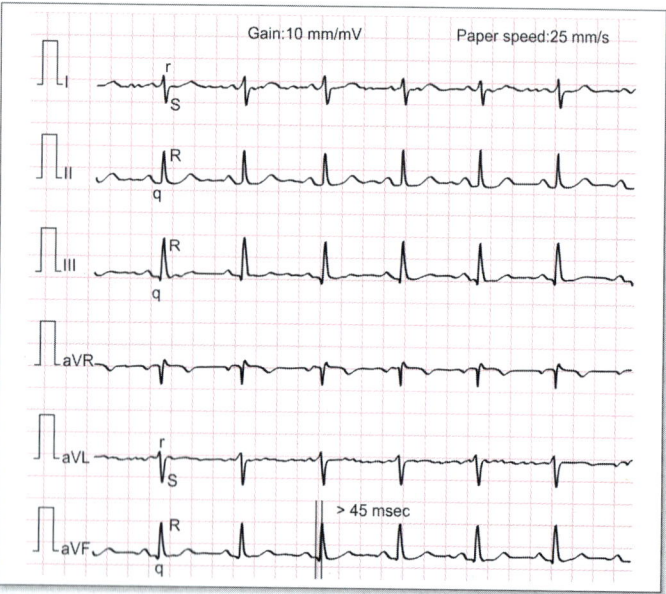

Fig. 10.10 ECG showing LPFB

- LAFB features - qR complexes in leads I and aVL and rS complexes in II, III, and aVF (Fig. 10.11).

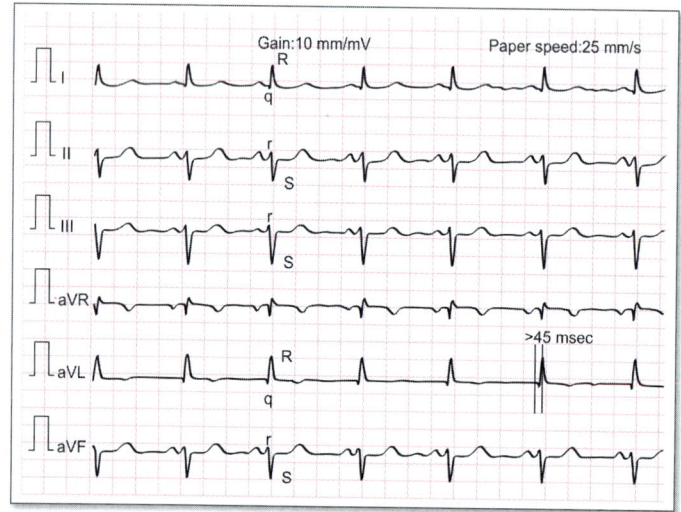

Fig. 10.11 ECG showing LAFB

Causes of Fascicular Blocks (LAFB and LPFB)

- Ischemic heart disease
- Degenerative disease
- Myocarditis
- Hyperkalaemia
- Cardiomyopathy
- Amyloidosis
- Hypertension

Management

- Assess for association with RBBB
- Monitor ECG
- Usually asymptomatic with isolated fascicular block but with bifascicular blocks there may be transient syncope in patient.

Practice Questions

1. **Identify the rhythm**
   a. First degree AV Block
   b. Mobitz type I (Wenchebach's)
   c. Mobitz type II
   d. Third degree AV Block

2. **Identify the rhythm**
   a. First degree AV Block
   b. Second degree AV Block
   c. Third degree AV block
   d. 2:1 block

3. **Identify the rhythm**
   a. First degree AV Block
   b. Second degree type I AV Block
   c. Second degree type II AV Block
   d. Third degree AV block

4. **Identify the rhythm**
   a. Second degree AV Block
   b. Left bundle Branch block
   c. Right bundle branch block
   d. Complete heart block

5. **Identify the rhythm**
   a. Second degree AV Block
   b. Left bundle Branch block
   c. Right bundle branch block
   d. Complete heart block

Answers

1. b   2. d   3. d   4. b   5. c

ECG Changes in Electrolyte Disturbances

Chapter 11

INTRODUCTION

- Normal cardiac action potential may be altered by electrolyte imbalance due to changes in intracellular and extracellular electrolyte concentrations.
- Most common and clinically most relevant electrolyte imbalances concern potassium, calcium and magnesium. These electrolytes may be life threatening.

ELECTROCARDIOGRAM AND POTASSIUM (TABLE 11.1)

ECG Changes due to Hyperkalaemia

- **Mild hyperkalaemia (potassium 5.5-6.5 mEq/L)**
  - Pointed T wave (narrow and tall)
- **Moderate hyperkalaemia (potassium 6.5-8 mEq/L)**
  - Pointed T wave (more pronounced)
  - Wide P wave, decreased P wave amplitude
  - Prolonged PR interval ST segment may occur in V1-V3
- **Severe hyperkalaemia (potassium>8 mEq/L)**
  - More pronounced ECG changes mentioned previously
  - Wide QRS complex
  - Fusion of QRS complex with T wave forming sine wave which may precede ventricular fibrillation

ECG Changes in Hypokalaemia

- Wide T wave with lower amplitude
- T wave inversion in severe hypokalaemia
- ST segment depression
- Increase in P wave amplitude, duration and PR interval
- Prominent U wave (best seen in lead V2-V3). In case of severe hypokalaemia, U wave may become larger than the T wave.

- May lead to acquired long QT syndrome and predisposes to polymorphic or monomorphic ventricular tachycardia.
- May potentiates the pro arrhythmis effect of digoxin.

Table 11.1 Comparative analysis of ECG and potassium level in blood

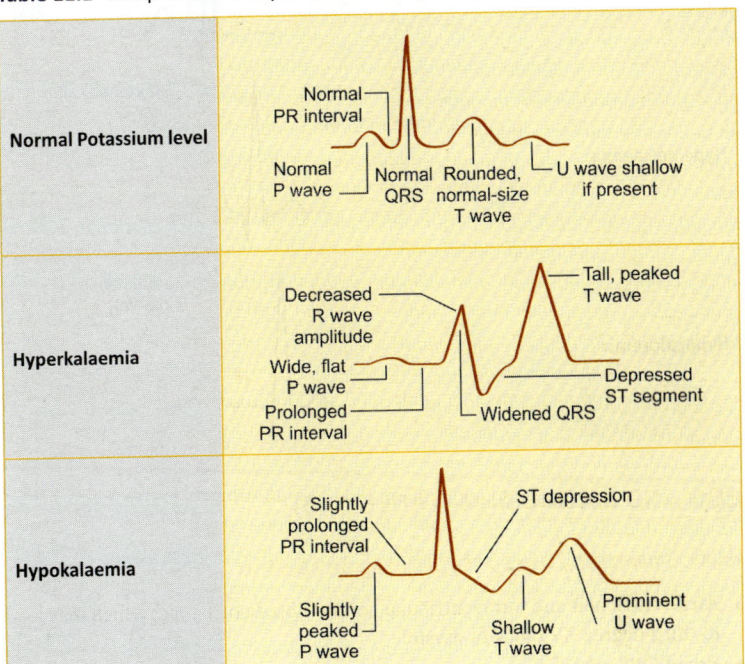

ECG AND CALCIUM (TABLE 11.2)

ECG Changes Due to Hypercalcaemia

- Shortened QT interval
- Lengthened QRS duration
- Bradycardia may occur

ECG Changes Due to Hypocalcaemia

- Lengthened QT interval
- Shortened QRS duration

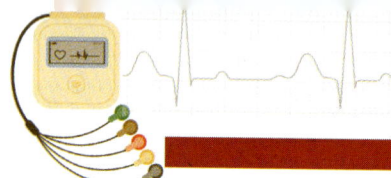
Table 11.2 Comparative analysis of ECG and calcium level in blood

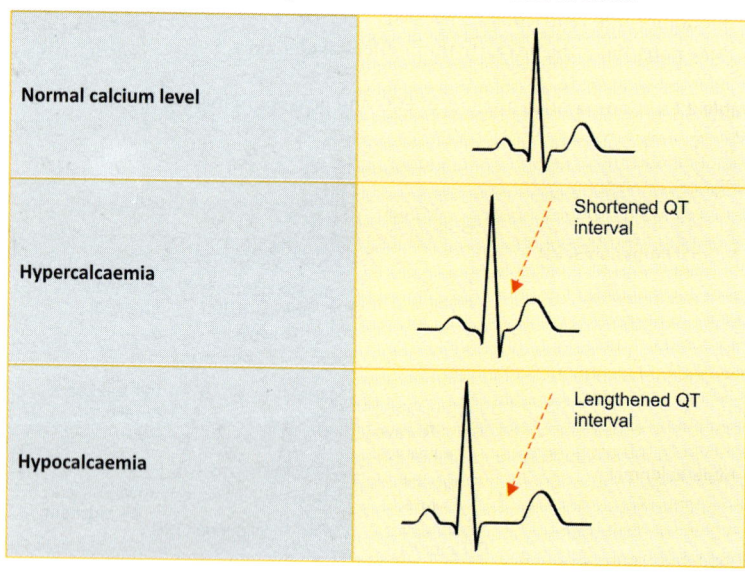

Normal calcium level	
Hypercalcaemia	Shortened QT interval
Hypocalcaemia	Lengthened QT interval

ECG AND MAGNESIUM (TABLE 11.3)

ECG Changes Due to Hypermagnesaemia

- Atrioventricular and intraventricular conduction disturbances which may lead to third degree AV block or asystole
- Broad QRS complex
- Prolonged PR interval

ECG Changes Due to Hypomagnesaemia

- Hypomagnesaemia may predispose to supraventricular and ventricular tachyarrhythmias and also potentiates the Proarrhythmic effect of digoxin
- On ECG, Lengthened QT, broad and flattened T wave can be seen.
- It often co-exists with hypokalaemia.

Table 11.3 Comparative analysis of ECG and magnesium level in blood

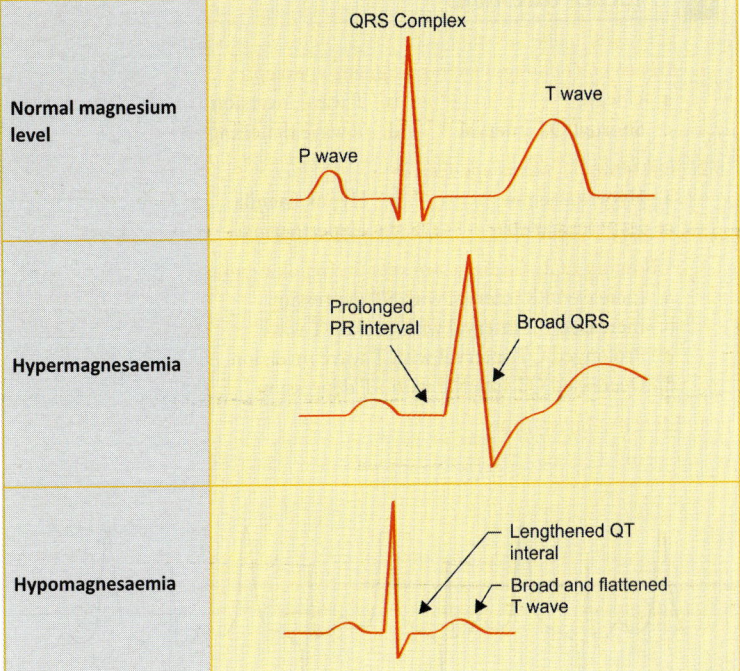

Normal magnesium level	QRS Complex, T wave, P wave
Hypermagnesaemia	Prolonged PR interval, Broad QRS
Hypomagnesaemia	Lengthened QT interal, Broad and flattened T wave

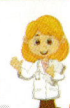

Must Know

Many arrhyhmias (discussed previously) are due to imbalances in electrolytes so always make sure to obtain serum electrolyte level of patients presenting with arrythmias.

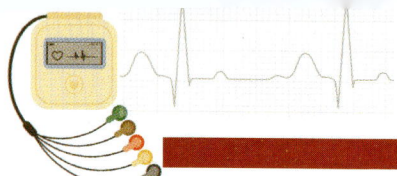
 Practice Questions

1. **All are ECG changes in hypokalaemia, except:**
   a. U wave   b. T wave inversion
   c. Shorten QT interval d. T wave flattening

2. **Tall tented T waves are seen in:**
   a. Hyperkalaemia   b. Hypokalaemia
   c. Hypercalcaemia   d. Hyperthermia

3. **Following ECG findings are seen in hypokalemia:**
   a. Increased PR interval with ST depression
   b. Increased PR interval with peaked T wave
   c. Prolonged QT interval with T wave inversion
   d. Decreased QT interval with ST depression

4. **Identify the rhythm:**

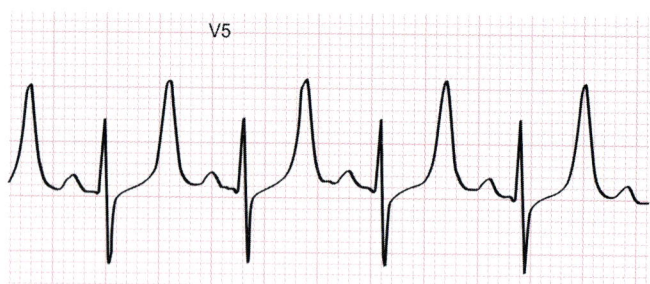

5. **QT interval is shortened in:**
   a. Hypocalcaemia   b. Hypophosphataemia
   c. Hypercalcaemia   d. Hypokalaemia

6. **Identify the rhythm:**

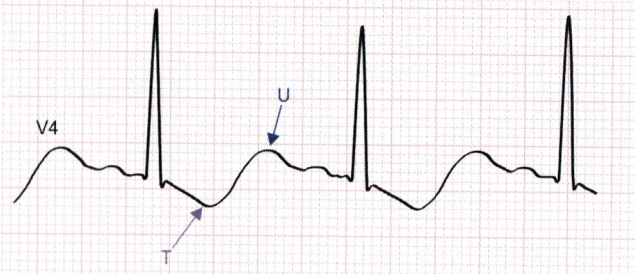

7. Identify the rhythm:

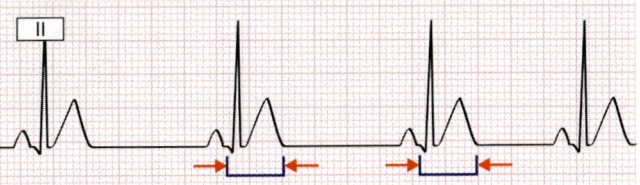

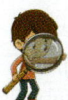
Answers

1. c
2. a
3. a
4. Hyperkalemia

5. c
6. Hypokalemia
7. Hypercalcemia

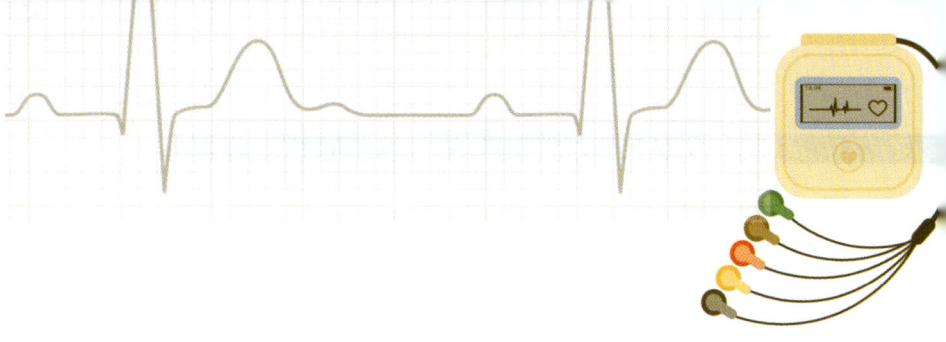

Annexures

PATIENT EDUCATION FOR ANTICOAGULATION THERAPY

Warfarin

- Explain the patient about reasons for starting anticoagulation therapy.
- Describe the mechanism of action of anticoagulant and possible side effects of the medication, in a language easily understood by the patient.
- Patient needs to inform all health care providers that he/she is on anticoagulants.
- The patient does not need to avoid foods rich in vitamin K such as spinach, broccoli etc., but must not take much.
- Advice to:
  - Take the medication at same time everyday.
  - Get PT/INR checked periodically as advised. In a patient on anticoagulants, target INR valve is 2-3, whereas patients on mechanical valves it is 2.5-3.5. Explain that increased INR makes patient to bleed easily.
  - Avoid situations that could lead to trauma such as contact sports, use of straight razor, vigorous brushing of teeth, cutting vegetables or fruits, using needles etc.
  - Use soft brush to prevent gum bleeding.
  - Not to take supplemental vitamin K.
  - Always carry identification card which clearly shows that patient is on anticoagulants.
  - Not to stop the drug abruptly.
  - Not to take alcohol.
- Explain the signs which may require immediate medical attention, such as:
  - Any bleeding that does not stop after a reasonable amount of time (usually 10-15 minutes).
  - Unusual bleeding from gums, throat, skin or nose or heavy menstrual bleeding.
  - Severe headache or stomach pain.

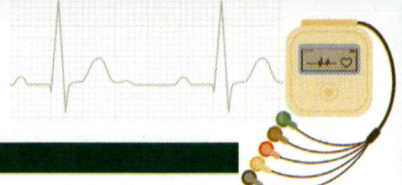

- Blood in vomiting, urine or stool. Presence of black, tarry stool.
- Cold, blue or painful feet.
- Weakness, dizziness or mental status changes.

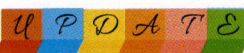

Apart from Warfarin, newer anticoagulants are also available now a days. Patients do not need to monitor their PT/INR level(s) with these anticoagulants. Few examples are: Dabigatran. Rivaroxaban and Apixaban.

Difference between Defibrillation and Cardioversion

Sl. No.	Defibrillation	Cardioversion
1.	It is done in emergency.	It is an elective procedure.
2	Client remains unconscious.	Consent has to be obtained from the patient for Cardioversion
3	Used if patient has ventricular fibrillation or pulseless ventricular tachycardia.	Used in most of the arrythmias except ventricular fibrillation and pulseless ventricular tachycardia.
4	High energy shock is delivered.	Low energy shock is delivered.
5	Shock given during defibrillation is unsynchronized	Shock is synchronized with QRS complex.
6	Associated with more damage to myocardium.	Associated with less damage to myocardium.
7	Anticoagulation is not needed.	Anticoagulation is needed.
8	Sedatives are not required.	Sedatives are required.

DIFFERENCES BETWEEN MONOPHASIC AND BIPHASIC DEFIBRILLATOR

Sl. No.	Monophasic Defibrillator	Biphasic Defibrillator
1.	In this, the current travels only in one direction- from one paddle to the other.	In this, the current travels in two directions, first towards the positive paddle and than reverses and goes back which occurs several times.
2.	Higher amount of energy is required to deliver the shock. Usually 360 Joules.	Lower amount of energy is required to deliver the shock. Usually 120-200 Joules
3.	Associated with more burns	Associated with lesser burns

Contd...

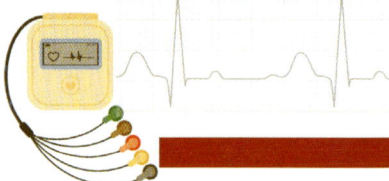
Sl. No.	Monophasic Defibrillator	Biphasic Defibrillator
4.	Causes myocardial damage	Myocardial damage occurs to less extent
5.	Leads to more trauma	Trauma is less
6.	In monophasic shocks, the rate of first shock success in cardiac arrest due to a shockable rhythm is only 60%.	In biphasic shocks, first shock success rate in cardiac arrest due to a shockable rhythm is around 90%.

Monophasic	**Biphasic**
Current delivered in **one** direction	Current delivered in **two** direction

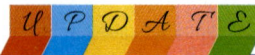

Nowadays Triphasic and Quadriphasic defibrillators are also available.

PATIENT EDUCATION FOR PATIENTS ON PERMANENT PACEMAKER (FIG. 1)

A pacemaker is an electronic device that provides electrical stimuli to the heart muscles.

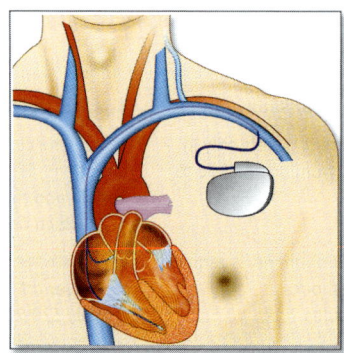

Fig. 1 Pacemaker

PATIENT EDUCATION

- Teach patient to check own pulse for one minute daily preferebly on the same site and maintain the diary for the same.
- Report slowing on the pulse less than the set rate.
- Report signs and symptoms as palpitations, fatigue, dizziness and frequent hiccups.
- Wear identification bracelet and carry a pacemaker identity card.

Site Care

- Always wash your hands before touching the wound.
- Wear loose fitting clothes around pacemeker.
- Do not wear clothes that rub on the wound for 2-3 weeks.
- Watch for sign and symptoms of infection like fever,
- Keep incision site clean and dry, not to scrub the site. After 4-5 days of pacemaker insertion shower may be taken, be careful to pat dry the area.

Electromagnetic Inference

- Explain that high energy radar, TV and radio transmitters, antitheft devices and airpost security alarms may affect the pacemaker function.
- Ask to be hand searched after showing your card.
- Most security gates at airports and stores are OK. But do not stand near these devices for long periods. Pacemaker may set off alarms.
- Teach patient to move 4-6 meters away from the source and check pulse, it should return to normal.

Cell Phone

- Do not put it in a pocket on the same side of body as pacemaker.
- When using the cell phone, hold it to your ear on the opposite side of your body.

Follow up

Patients with pacemaker should routinely visit the cardiologist as per the planned follow up visits.

ECG showing pacing spikes with pacemaker is depicted in Figure 2.

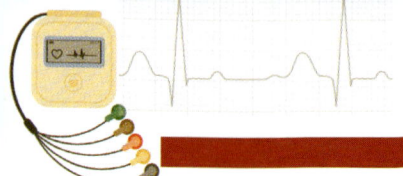

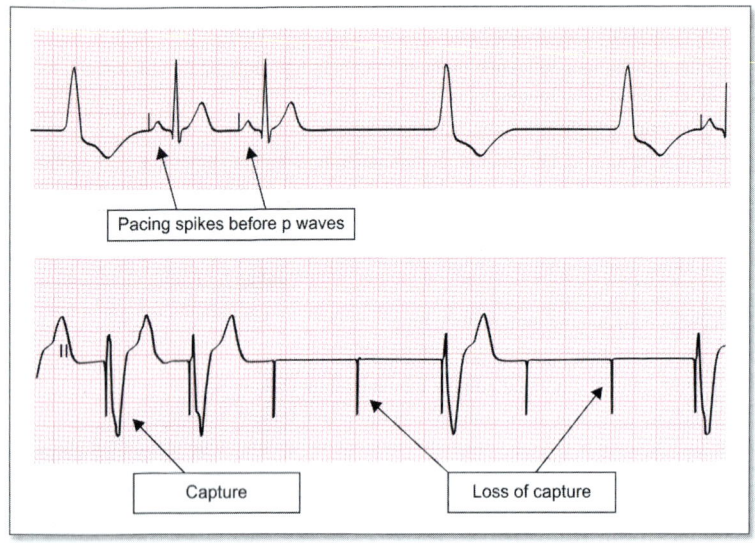

Pacing spikes before p waves

Capture

Loss of capture

Fig. 2 ECG showing pacing spikes with pacemaker

AMERICAN HEART ASSOCIATION'S GUIDELINES FOR
CARDIOPULMONARY RESUSCITATION

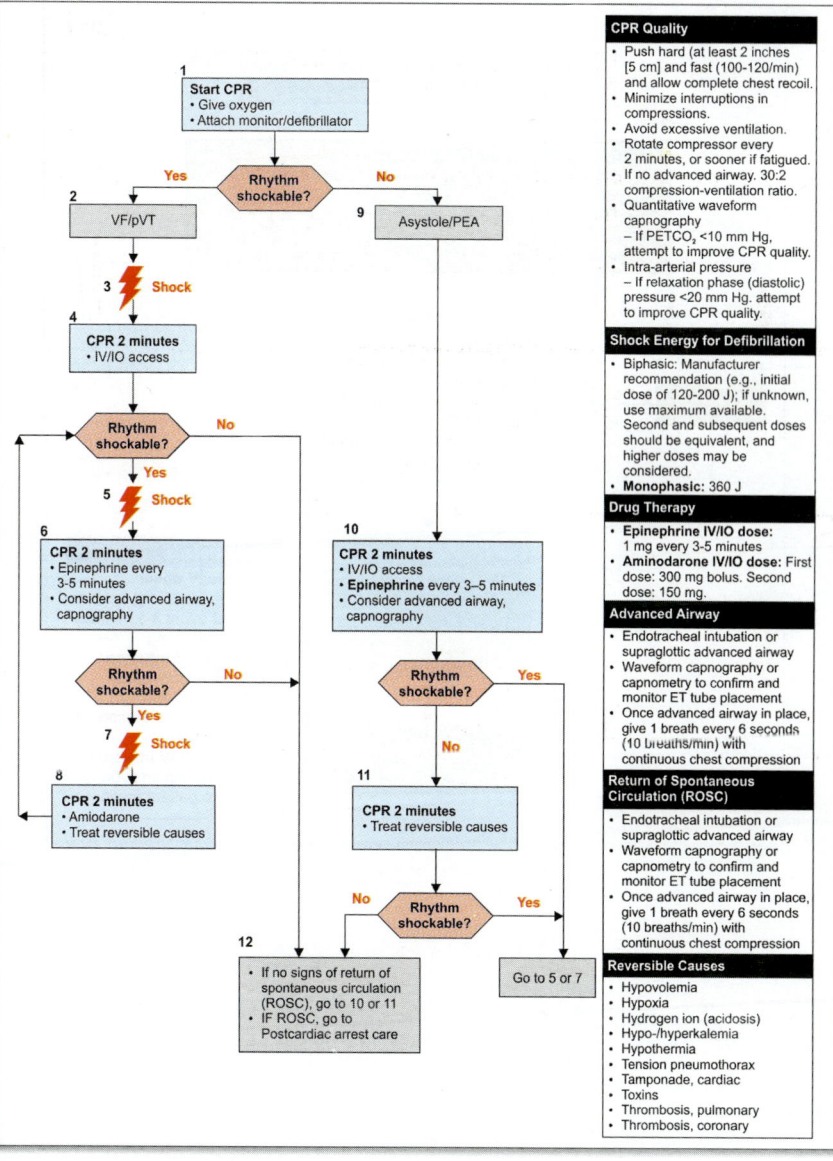

AMERICAN HEART ASSOCIATION'S GUIDELINES FOR BRADYCARDIA

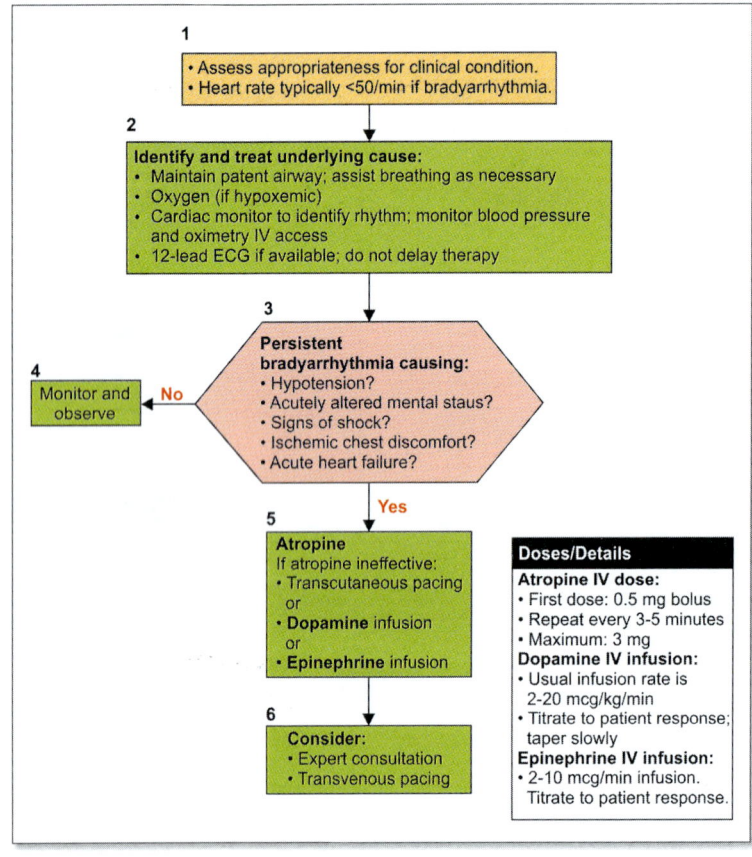

1
- Assess appropriateness for clinical condition.
- Heart rate typically <50/min if bradyarrhythmia.

2

Identify and treat underlying cause:
- Maintain patent airway; assist breathing as necessary
- Oxygen (if hypoxemic)
- Cardiac monitor to identify rhythm; monitor blood pressure and oximetry IV access
- 12-lead ECG if available; do not delay therapy

3

Persistent bradyarrhythmia causing:
- Hypotension?
- Acutely altered mental staus?
- Signs of shock?
- Ischemic chest discomfort?
- Acute heart failure?

4

No

Monitor and observe

Yes

5

Atropine
If atropine ineffective:
- Transcutaneous pacing
or
- **Dopamine** infusion
or
- **Epinephrine** infusion

6

Consider:
- Expert consultation
- Transvenous pacing

Doses/Details

Atropine IV dose:
- First dose: 0.5 mg bolus
- Repeat every 3-5 minutes
- Maximum: 3 mg

Dopamine IV infusion:
- Usual infusion rate is 2-20 mcg/kg/min
- Titrate to patient response; taper slowly

Epinephrine IV infusion:
- 2-10 mcg/min infusion. Titrate to patient response.

AMERICAN HEART ASSOCIATION'S GUIDELINES FOR TACHYCARDIA

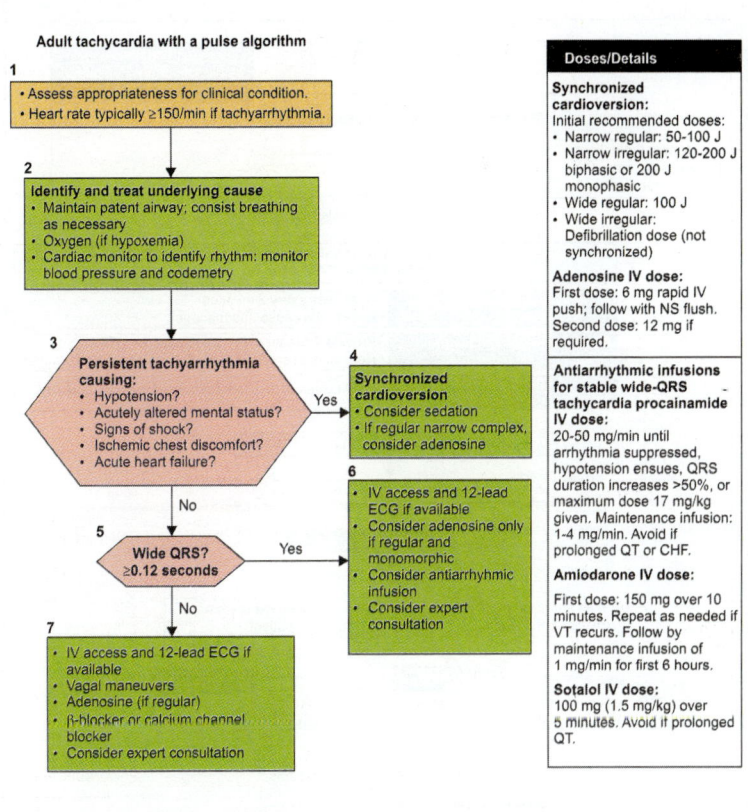

Adult tachycardia with a pulse algorithm

1
- Assess appropriateness for clinical condition.
- Heart rate typically ≥150/min if tachyarrhythmia.

2
Identify and treat underlying cause
- Maintain patent airway; consist breathing as necessary
- Oxygen (if hypoxemia)
- Cardiac monitor to identify rhythm: monitor blood pressure and codemetry

3
Persistent tachyarrhythmia causing:
- Hypotension?
- Acutely altered mental status?
- Signs of shock?
- Ischemic chest discomfort?
- Acute heart failure?

Yes →

4
Synchronized cardioversion
- Consider sedation
- If regular narrow complex, consider adenosine

No ↓

5
Wide QRS?
≥0.12 seconds

Yes →

6
- IV access and 12-lead ECG if available
- Consider adenosine only if regular and monomorphic
- Consider antiarrhythmic infusion
- Consider expert consultation

No ↓

7
- IV access and 12-lead ECG if available
- Vagal maneuvers
- Adenosine (if regular)
- β-blocker or calcium channel blocker
- Consider expert consultation

Doses/Details

Synchronized cardioversion:
Initial recommended doses:
- Narrow regular: 50-100 J
- Narrow irregular: 120-200 J biphasic or 200 J monophasic
- Wide regular: 100 J
- Wide irregular: Defibrillation dose (not synchronized)

Adenosine IV dose:
First dose: 6 mg rapid IV push; follow with NS flush. Second dose: 12 mg if required.

Antiarrhythmic infusions for stable wide-QRS tachycardia procainamide IV dose:
20-50 mg/min until arrhythmia suppressed, hypotension ensues, QRS duration increases >50%, or maximum dose 17 mg/kg given. Maintenance infusion: 1-4 mg/min. Avoid if prolonged QT or CHF.

Amiodarone IV dose:
First dose: 150 mg over 10 minutes. Repeat as needed if VT recurs. Follow by maintenance infusion of 1 mg/min for first 6 hours.

Sotalol IV dose:
100 mg (1.5 mg/kg) over 5 minutes. Avoid if prolonged QT.

COMPREHENSIVE CARDIOPULMONARY LIFE SUPPORT (CCLS) ALGORITHM BY INDIAN RESUSCITATION COUNCIL

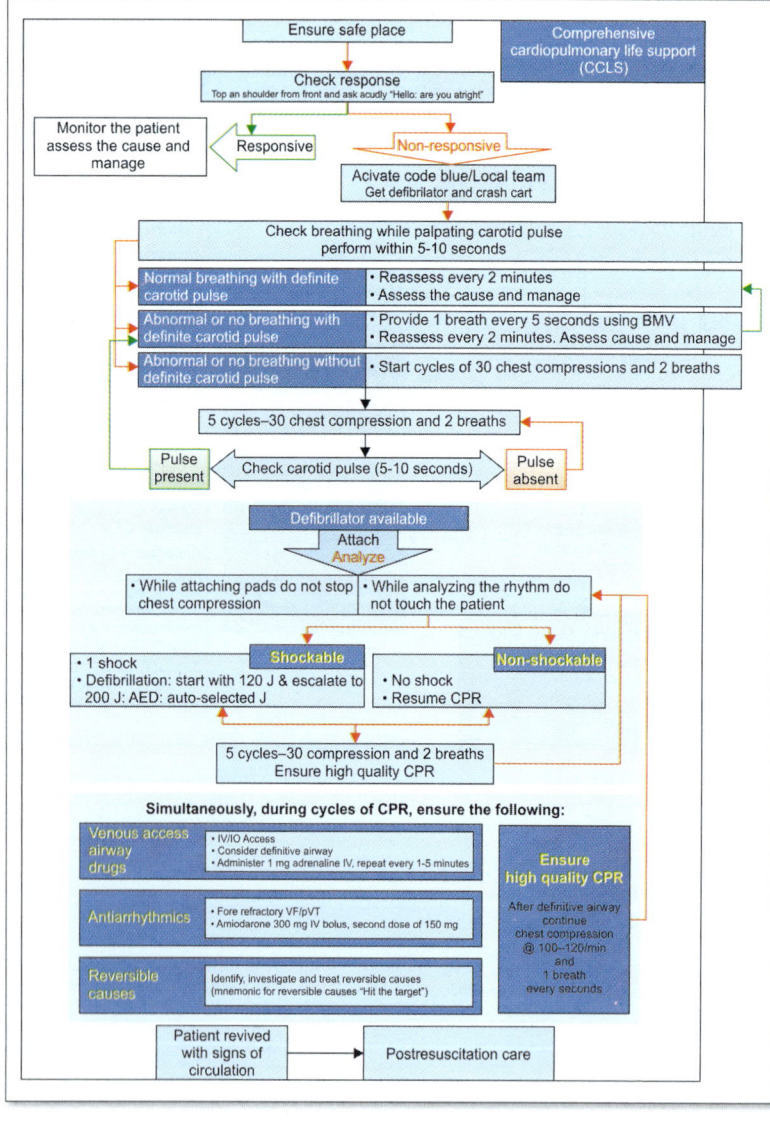

NURSING PROCESS APPLIED FOR THE PATIENT HAVING HEART BLOCK

Decreased Cardiac Output

Nursing Assessment

- Decreased level of consciousness
- Syncope
- Shortness of breath
- Light headedness
- Dizziness
- Fatigue
- Chest discomfort
- Palpitations
- Pale and cool skin

History

Obtain a health history to identify any previous occurrences of decreased cardiac output such as light headedness, syncope (fainting), dizziness, fatigue, chest discomfort, and palpitations.

Assess for any **co-existing conditions**—any previous or newly diagnosed heart disease or any other systemic illness or co-morbidity like diabetes, hypertension, etc.

Assess **medication history** (especially those which may decrease HR like digoxin, beta blockers, etc.) or any medication taken by patient himself (over the counter drug) or any herb.

Assess for **sign of shock**—hypotension, cool and pale skin, altered mental status, decreased urine output.

Nursing Diagnosis

Decreased cardiac output related to altered heart rhythm as evidenced by loss of consciousness, light headedness, dizziness, chest discomfort, palpitations and cool peripheries.

Planning

To achieve and maintain adequate cardiac output, cerebral and peripheral tissue perfusion.

Nursing Interventions

- Assess level of consciousness and sensorium.
- Assess SpO_2 using pulse oximetry

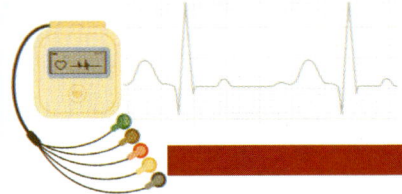

- Monitor vital signs, palpate pulses, note significant variations in the blood pressure.
- Obtain 12 lead ECG and interpret the type of block.
- Check changes in skin color and temperature.
- Monitor urine output.
- Auscultate heart sounds, noting rate, rhythm, presence of extra heartbeats, or any dropped beats.
- If the **patient is hemodynamically stable**—assess and maintain—Airway, Breathing and Circulation.
- If **patient is not hemodynamically stable,** i.e. hypoxemic, decreasing oxygen saturation (SpO_2), altered mental status, shortness of breath etc.—maintain airway by endotracheal intubation and prepare the patient for emergent temporary pacing (**transcutaneous pacing**).
- If patient is conscious and needs urgent pacing, consider sedation if time allows, and if sedation is available before the procedure.
- A nurse should keep the articles arranged required for the pacing.

Evaluation

Expected patient outcomes may include:
- Maintain cardiac output
- Demonstrates heart rate, blood pressure, respiratory rate and level of consciousness within normal ranges
- Demonstrates no or decreased episodes of dysrhythmia

NURSING CARE WITH TEMPORARY TRANSCUTANEOUS PACING

In patient with heart block (2° or 3° blocks) pacing is required. Temporary pacing—catheter insertion may be performed at bed side or in the cardiac catheterization lab.

Before Catheter Insertion

- Explain the procedure to the patient and family and obtain **informed written consent.**
- Part preparation should be done.
- Insert the IV line if not present and if already present check the patency of the intravenous line or heparin lock.
- Collect all the articles and also have emergency equipment available (crash cart).
- Check the working condition of all the equipment required for the procedure and ensure that electrical equipment are properly grounded and electrically safe.

- Sedate the patient if necessary or as prescribed.
- Attach the ECG electrodes and machine to the patient

During Cathter Insertion

- Monitor cardiac rhythm closely
- Check vitals, specifically blood pressure and HR every 10–15 minutes or more frequently and also record the fluctuations.
- Give emotional support to the patient.

After Catheter Insertion

- Obtain a 12 lead ECG for baseline determination of catheter position
- Obtain a chest radiograph, lateral if possible to determine catheter position.
- Assess the site of pacing catheter insertion for infection (redness, discharge, tenderness, warmth at area or swelling), bleeding or hematoma.
- Selectively restrict the patient's movement to prevent pacer wire dislodgment.
- Enforce bed rest initially and also inform the patient the need for the same.
- Make sure all the electrical instruments or devices used nearby patient should be properly grounded to prevent electrical interference and shock to the patient.
- Assess pacemaker spikes in the ECG and its relation to the ECG complexes to determine pacemaker functioning.
- Administer the prescribed medications and analgesics.
- Check and keep all the connections secure.
- Assess the electrolytes level of the patient especially serum potassium.
- Support the patient emotionally and clarify the queries by patient and relatives.
- Document the following:
  - Date and time of insertion
  - Type of wire inserted and location of insertion
  - Whether the pacer is on or off.
  - Rate setting of pacer.
  - Threshold level and mA setting
  - AV interval if AV sequential mode is used.

HEART BLOCK – EASY TO REMEMBER

Heart block is a condition in which electrical impulses are either delayed or completely blocked at AV node (Chapter 10).

This annexure is an easy way to remember Heart block in a story format of husband, wife and a counsellor.

Wife = P Wave
Husband = QRS Complex
Pacer = Counselling

Normal Sinus Rhythm
The wife (P wave) waits at home for the husband (QRS).
The husband (QRS) comes home on time every night.

PR Interval is less than 0.20 seconds (One large block on the EKG paper or 3 to 5 small boxes), there is one P wave per QRS complex, and the rhythm is regular.

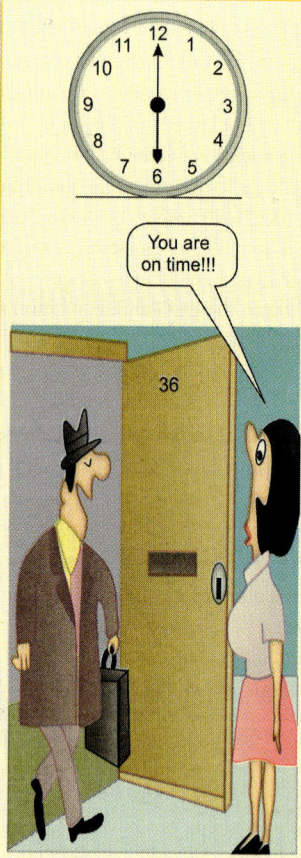

1st Degree AV Block
The wife (P wave) is waiting at home. **The Husband (QRS) comes home late every night, but he always comes home, and it is the same time, every night.**

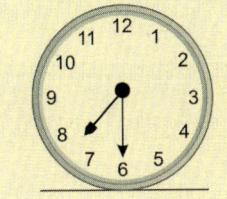

Impulse is held/ delayed at AV node, and PR Interval is greater than 0.20 seconds, or one large box on the EKG paper (>5 small boxes)

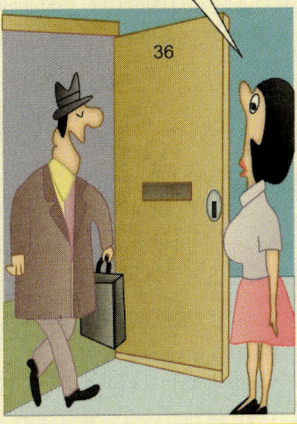

2nd Degree Block, Type 1 ("Wenckebach")
The wife (P wave) is waiting at home. The husband (QRS) comes home **later and later every night until one night he doesn't come home at all.**

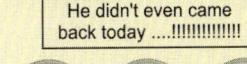

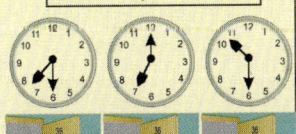

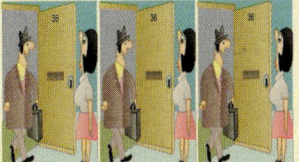

PR interval will become greater and greater until there will be a dropped QRS complex and there are two consecutive P waves, after which the pattern will restart.

Note: Husband (QRS) must come home at least 2 nights in a row to see this pattern.
It may require counselling (pacing)

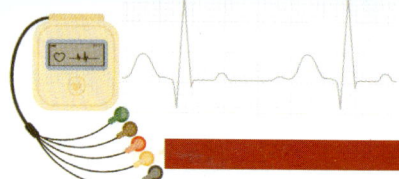

2nd Degree Block, Type 2

The wife (P wave) is waiting at home. **Sometimes the husband (QRS) comes home, sometimes he doesn't.** When he does come home, it's always at the same time.

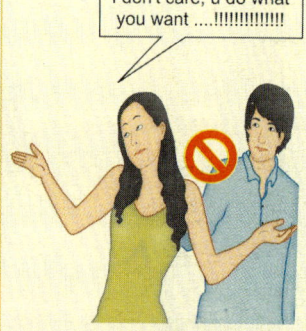

Note: This is usually more serious than Type I, and will sometimes require counselling (pacing).

PR and R to R intervals will remain consistent, but there will be "missing" QRS complexes.

3rd Degree AV Block

Wife (P wave) is no longer waiting at home. She and her husband (QRS) are now on separate schedules, have no concern to one another, and are no longer talking. **Each spouse (P wife and QRS husband) has a regular, individual schedule.**

I don't care, u do what you want ....!!!!!!!!!!!!!!!

Note: This frequently requires Counselling in the form of a temporary or permanent pacer.

Atrial depolarisation will continue with P waves in a "ventricular standstill" while the ventricles (QRS) are depolarising in an idioventricular rhythm – both will be regular, but will be uncoordinated or not-synchronized